Contents

About the author

Stanley Mutsatsa is a former Course Leader in Medication Management at Kings College, Institute of Psychiatry, London. He is currently a Senior Lecturer in the Faculty of Health and Social Care at London South Bank University.

Contributor: Chapter 1

Suzanne Waugh is Learning Skills tutor at the University of Salford. Her background is in both Archaeology and Psychology, and she currently runs the university's study skills programme. Suzanne is also a qualified adult numeracy teacher, and is developing numeracy provision for student nurses.

Acknowledgements

The authors and publisher would like to thank the following for permission to reproduce copyright material:

Elsevier Ltd. for data in Table 3.1 (page 79), Stages of change and associated patient characteristics and possible interventions, reproduced from Chapman, KR, Walker, L, Cluley, S and Fabbri, L (2000) Improving patient compliance with asthma therapy, *Respiratory Medicine* 94 (1): 2–9.

Every effort has been made to trace all copyright holders within the book, but if any have been inadvertently overlooked the publisher will be pleased to make the necessary arrangements at the first opportunity.

A special thanks to Simon Thistle for the artistic contribution and advice.

Medicines Management in Mental Health Nursing

Stanley Mutsatsa

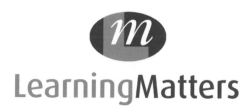

LearningMatters

First published in 2011 by Learning Matters Ltd

British Library Cataloguing in Publication Data
A CIP record for this book is available from the British Library

ISBN: 978 0 85725 049 0

This book is also available in the following ebook formats:

Adobe ebook: 978 0 85725 051 3
ePUB ebook: 978 0 85725 050 6
Kindle: 978 0 85725 0 520

The right of Stanley Mutsatsa and Suzanne Waugh to be identified as the authors of this Work has been asserted by them in accordance with the Copyright, Designs and Patents Act 1988.

Cover and text design by Toucan Design
Project management by Diana Chambers
Typeset by Kelly Winter
Printed and bound in Great Britain by Short Run Press Ltd, Exeter, Devon

Learning Matters Ltd
20 Cathedral Yard
Exeter EX1 1HB
Tel: 01392 215560
E-mail: info@learningmatters.co.uk
www.learningmatters.co.uk

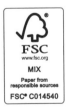

Introduction

About this book

This book is aimed at supporting pre-registration mental health nursing students to meet the NMC competencies for medicines management. It is structured around the NMC Essential Skills Cluster for Medicines Management to prepare the student for a formative and summative assessment for entry into the register of mental health nurses. Although the book is primarily aimed at nursing students at the pre-registration level of training, it will also serve as a useful reference guide for post-registration nurses. A link between theory and practice is made explicit and the book is written in a style that is easy to understand, offering academic challenge without diluting academic integrity.

Why is Medicines Management important for mental health nurses?

Despite the demonstrable importance of psychotropic medication, existing evidence suggests that registered nurses' knowledge and skills in medicines management is deficient. Nurses have felt that their practice is hampered by a lack of appropriate educational preparation. In particular, they cite poor knowledge of psychopharmacology as one of the main reasons for a lack of confidence in their role.

The NMC Essential Skills Clusters (ESCs) were developed as an outcome of the review of nurses' fitness to practise at the point of registration. The ESCs aim to address some of the concerns that were raised around skill deficits in nurses, and medicines management is one specific area identified. As from September 2008 it has been a mandatory requirement that all student nurses demonstrate competency in drug administration and calculation at two progression points and prior to registration. This textbook meets the requirements for the application of mental health nursing's specific competencies in medicines management.

Book structure

The book has twelve chapters. Chapter 1 covers basic calculations likely to be encountered in medicines management. Chapter 2 covers the legal and ethical aspects of medicines management in mental health nursing, legislation pertaining to medicines management, ethics and account-ability.

Chapter 3 covers issues relating to the therapeutic alliance. These include the health belief model, the self-regulatory model, the problem of adherence to medication, factors that influence adherence, service barriers to adherence, decision-making capacity and the use of concordance skills to promote medication adherence.

Chapter 4 provides the necessary baseline knowledge of anatomy and physiology of the brain. It also forms the basis for an understanding of how psychotropic medications work.

Chapters 5 to 10 cover the management and treatment of various mental health problems: depression, bipolar disorder, psychosis, dementias, anxiety states and substance misuse disorders. In these chapters, we cover knowledge of the main clinical features and differential diagnosis of each condition before discussing specific treatment and management options. Each chapter outlines the common errors to avoid during treatment and management, and also summarises how to inform the patient.

Chapter 11 deals with drug interactions and the issues of pharmacodynamics and pharmacokinetics, including the role of race and ethnicity in drug interactions, which requires special consideration. Chapter 12 deals with the role of the multidisciplinary team in medicines management, record keeping, storage of medicines and administration.

Learning features

Activities

Throughout the book you will find activities in the text that will help you to make sense of, and learn about, the material being presented. All the activities require you to take a break from reading the text, think through the issues presented and carry out some independent study, possibly using the internet. Where appropriate, there are outline answers presented at the end of each chapter, and these will help you to understand more fully your own reflections and independent study. Remember, academic study will always require independent work; attending lectures will never be enough to be successful on your programme, and these activities will help to deepen your knowledge and understanding of the issues under scrutiny and give you practice at working on your own.

Case studies and scenarios

Within each chapter there are case studies that describe real-life situations from the practice environment. The case studies have been included so that you may further understand the material being presented. You may wish to discuss and reflect on the case studies with senior students, as they may have experienced similar situations and could provide valuable insights through their experience.

Scenarios are presented to find a fictitious but realistic perspective on the information being discussed. These have been included so that you may develop the skill of thinking about issues from a number of different viewpoints. For this reason, some of the scenarios require you to put yourself in another person's shoes, considering how and why you would react to a given situation.

There are explanations in the Glossary for words in **bold** in the text.

Chapter 1
Drug calculations

Suzanne Waugh

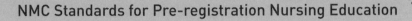
NMC Standards for Pre-registration Nursing Education

This chapter will address the following competencies:

Domain 3: Nursing practice and decision-making

6. All nurses must practise safely by being aware of the correct use, limitations and hazards of common interventions, including nursing activities, treatments, and the use of medical devices and equipment. The nurse must be able to evaluate their use, report any concerns promptly through appropriate channels and modify care where necessary to maintain safety. They must contribute to the collection of local and national data and formulation of policy on risks, hazards and adverse outcomes.

NMC Essential Skills Clusters

This chapter will address the following ESCs:

Cluster: Medicines management

33. People can trust the newly registered graduate nurse to correctly and safely undertake medicines calculations.

By the first progression point:

1. Is competent in basic medicines calculations relating to: tablets and capsules; liquid medicines; injections including: unit dose, sub and multiple unit dose, SI unit conversion.

By entry to the register:

2. Is competent in the process of medication-related calculation in nursing field involving: tablets and capsules; liquid medicines; injections.

Chapter aims

By the end of this chapter, you should be able to:

*   use the 'four rules' (addition, subtraction, multiplication and division) to carry out a range of calculations, including with decimals;

- convert between different SI units;
- calculate how many tablets or how much liquid is needed to fill a prescription;
- use drug calculation formulae to answer more complex questions about the amount of a drug required.

Introduction

How often do you use maths skills in your everyday life? From working out whether you have been given the right change in a shop, to checking whether your payslip is correct, maths is an integral part of our daily existence. You need maths in order to work out which special offer represents the best value in the supermarket, and how much your friend owes you when they have offered to go halves in a restaurant. Despite this, many people are not confident with the numeracy skills required for these kinds of tasks, and many have developed a fear of maths by the time they reach adulthood.

As a mental health nurse, you will need good numeracy skills in many aspects of your job. Take the example of Joanne Evans, a newly qualified nurse, who miscalculated the amount of insulin her patient needed. She injected the patient, 85-year-old Margaret Thomas of Pontypool in Wales, with ten times the required dose. By the time Evans had realised her mistake several hours later, Margaret Thomas had died (Stokes, 2009). Unfortunately, many examples such as this exist in every branch of nursing. Lomas (2009) reports that, in mental health nursing alone, the National Patient Safety Agency (NPSA) received 7,419 medication error reports between October 2007 and September 2008. Many of these were thought to be due to calculation errors, and it is 'highly likely' that many more incidents occur each year but are not reported (Lomas, 2009).

Miscalculations can clearly lead to serious health complications or even death for patients, and yet they are preventable human errors. From weighing patients to calculating how many tablets or how much syrup is required, accuracy is vital and mistakes can have devastating consequences. Many nurses and student nurses struggle with numeracy, and recently there has been a great deal of research into the possible reasons for and consequences of this (Jukes and Gilchrist, 2006; Weeks et al, 2000). This chapter takes you through the basic mathematics skills you will need in order to carry out your day-to-day duties. It looks at the mathematical processes themselves, and at how to apply these to real situations involving medicine administration.

Using calculators and estimating answers

Case study

Bill was prescribed diazepam suspension 10mg. Kirsty , a registered nurse, checked the diazepam syrup bottle and noted that the label said 'Diazepam suspension, 2mg/ml'. She used a calculator to determine how many

continued . . .

> *millilitres of suspension she needed to administer and concluded that it was 20ml, which she administered to Bill. The correct dose should have been 5ml.*

Although you may feel quite comfortable with using a calculator, it is vital that you understand the mathematics you are using and can work out answers without relying on one. There may not always be a calculator to hand, and although they may save you time and allow you to check your answer quickly, you need to understand what you are calculating rather than simply putting numbers into a machine. There will always be another nurse with whom you can check your answers; however, you should not be relying on their grasp of numeracy but on your own. Every nurse needs to be able to work medicine doses out by themselves, competently and reasonably quickly.

It is also worth mentioning estimation at this point, because you will inevitably need to use your judgement when calculating drug doses – does the answer you have come up with look reasonable? Most tablets, for example, are manufactured in a variety of strengths and you may not find one that is exactly the strength you require. Maybe you will need to give the patient three of the tablets you have in stock. However, if you have calculated the dose and found that you need to give the patient 30 of these tablets, you will hopefully be able to use your judgement and think that this seems like a rather large pile of tablets to be giving the patient in one dose. If you come up with an answer that seems unlikely or unreasonable, it is probable that you have made a mistake somewhere in your calculations. You will need to check your working out to find where you went wrong. If you have used a calculator, it is impossible to tell where the mistake has been made – in fact, many people assume that the answer must be correct because the calculator has provided it. Calculators cannot tell whether you have entered the correct numbers in the correct order, so it is vital that you understand the process you are going through in order to reach your answer, and that you can judge whether that answer seems reasonable.

You should also feel able to question the prescription itself if you feel that an error may have been made by the prescribing doctor – occasionally this does happen. Imagine that you have checked your working out several times and still come up with an answer of 30 tablets. Your colleague has also checked, and agrees with your answer. In this scenario, you will need to question the original prescription, as your own judgement should tell you that a dose of 30 tablets seems unlikely. Although you might feel nervous about questioning the doctor, it is extremely important for the patient's safety that you act upon any doubts about dosage that you may have.

How to use this chapter

You may feel that your numeracy skills are already good, and that you only need to skim through this section of the book. You might be competent in some areas, but not in others. It may be many years since you studied mathematics at school, or you may not have enjoyed it or found it difficult. It is natural to feel nervous about using a skill you are not completely confident with, particularly when accuracy is so important to your patients' health. Whatever your starting point, you should be able to find useful information and activities in this chapter that will help you to prepare yourself for the kinds of calculations you will need to perform as a nurse.

Activity 1.1	*Reflection*

Assess your own numeracy skills and how confident you feel with the following:

- adding and subtracting whole numbers;
- multiplication and division sums;
- understanding decimals: what they mean and adding, subtracting, multiplying and dividing decimals;
- converting between units, such as changing millilitres to litres;
- ratios and strengths of solutions;
- working out how many tablets or how much liquid is required in order to fill a prescription;
- how a patient's weight might affect the dose you are required to administer for some medicines.

As this activity is for self-assessment, no answer is provided.

As a nurse, you will need to be confident in all of the areas mentioned in the above activity. This chapter will look at each of them in turn.

What numbers are worth

Place value

The position of each **digit** within a larger number shows exactly what that digit is worth. You may remember using 'place value columns' at school, and these are useful tools when determining exactly what the value of each individual digit is. For example, if we take the number 482 and put it into a place value chart, it looks like this:

H	T	U
4	8	2

H stands for 'hundreds'   100
T stands for 'tens'   10
U stands for 'units' (which means 'ones')   1

So, we can see that the number 482 is made up of four 'hundreds', eight 'tens' and two 'units'.

The number 52,304 would fit into a place value chart like this:

TTh	Th	H	T	U
5	2	3	0	4

TTh stands for 'tens of thousands'   10,000
Th stands for 'thousands'   1000
H stands for 'hundreds'   100
T stands for 'tens'   10
U stands for 'units'   1

In this example, the number 52,304 is made up of five 'tens of thousands', two 'thousands', three 'hundreds', no tens and four 'units'. The zero in the 'tens' column is known as a place holder, and it is very important that we remember to include this zero – without it, many of the other digits would end up in the wrong columns and the number would represent a very different amount. Try the following activity to check how well you understand place value.

Activity 1.2

Work out the answers to the following questions.

1. Which number appears in the 'thousands' column of a place value chart for the number 562,103?
2. Write this number out in words: 24,086,079.
3. Write this number out in digits: three million, two hundred thousand, six hundred and fifty.
4. In the number 41,204,392, in which column of a place value chart would the digit 1 appear?
5. In the same number 41,204,392, in which column would the zero appear?

Answers to all activities can be found at the end of the chapter.

Decimals

Decimals or decimal fractions represent parts of whole numbers. We experience decimals every day, when we use money. Four pounds and twelve pence would be written as £4.12. The whole numbers in this case are pounds. Everything after the decimal point represents a small part of a whole number and everything before the decimal point represents a whole number, so in this case there are four whole units before the decimal point (the four pounds). In the same way as before, the number can be fitted into a place value chart in order to show the true values of the digits that appear after the decimal point:

U	.	1/10	1/100
4	.	1	2

1/10 means one 'tenth', or one out of ten.
1/100 means one 'hundredth', or one out of one hundred.

In order to work out exactly what the 1 and 2 represent, we need to look at the column headings. In this case, there is one 'tenth' of a whole, and two 'hundredths'. Imagine something has been divided into ten equal parts – each one is called a tenth. Using money, this means that a pound has been divided into ten 10p pieces, and we have one of those pieces. Similarly, a pound can also be divided into one hundred hundredths (pence or pennies), and we have two of them. Imagining our £4.12 laid out in front of you using these coins, you would have four pound coins, one ten pence coin and two pennies. It can often help to imagine money when dealing with decimals, to help you to understand the quantities you are dealing with. Look at the next example:

H	T	U	.	1/10	1/100	1/1000
3	4	6	.	9	2	3

The number 346.923 is made up of the following:

- three hundreds;
- four tens;
- six units;
- nine tenths;
- two hundredths;
- three thousandths.

You would say it as 'three hundred and forty-six point nine two three'.

Just as with whole numbers, decimal numbers sometimes require a place holder zero to show that there is nothing in one of the columns. Again, without this zero, the number would mean something quite different as some of the digits would be in the wrong columns. For example:

T	U	.	1/10	1/100
2	0	.	0	4

This number is 20.04 or twenty point zero four. It represents two tens, no units, no tenths and four hundredths. It may help to imagine this amount as money, £20.04. If you forgot to put the zero place holder in the units column, for example, the number would become £2.04, which is a very different amount to have in your pocket.

Activity 1.3

Answer the following questions.

1. Write 'fourteen pounds and three pence' out using digits in a place value chart.
2. What does the digit 6 represent in the number 128.46?
3. In which place value column does the digit 7 appear in the number 4.107?
4. Which of these numbers is bigger: 1.2 or 1.09?

Multiplying by 10, by 100 or by 1000

We know that $6 \times 10 = 60$. What is happening to the place value chart when we multiply 6 by 10?

T	U
	6

$\downarrow \times 10$

T	U
6	0

The 6 has moved one place to the left into the tens column, and a place holder zero has been written in the units column as there are no units. Similarly, we know that $2 \times 100 = 200$, but how does this look in a place value chart?

```
H    T    U
          2
              ↓ × 100
2    0    0
```

This time, the 2 has moved two places to the left into the hundreds column, and the tens and units columns now both have place holder zeros in them. Do you notice the pattern? There is one zero in 10, so when multiplying by 10 we need to move one place to the left. There are two zeros in 100, so when multiplying by 100 we move our digits two places to the left. There are three zeros in 1000, so if we multiply our original number by 1000, it will move three places to the left, and so on.

Activity 1.4

Try the following calculations.

1. 3×1000
2. 29×100
3. 86×10
4. 3462×100
5. 70×1000

This works in exactly the same way when multiplying decimals. For example, 7.6×10 would look like this:

```
T    U   .   1/10
     7   .   6
              ↓ × 10
7    6   .   0
```

The answer is 76 (you do not need to write 76.0).

Similarly, 29.027×100 would be:

```
Th   H    T    U   .   1/10   1/100   1/1000
          2    9   .   0      2       7
                                ↓ × 100
2    9    0    2   .   7
```

We have multiplied by 100, so everything has moved two columns to the left. The answer is 2902.7.

Activity 1.5

Try the following calculations:

1. 12.5×100
2. 349.04×10
3. 66.2×1000

Dividing by 10, by 100 or by 1000

We know that $70 \div 10 = 7$. Demonstrating this using a place value chart shows us that all digits have now moved one place to the right:

T   U
7   0
$\quad\quad \downarrow \div 10$
7

Dividing by 100 will mean that everything moves two places to the right, so $300 \div 100 = 3$, like this:

H   T   U
3   0   0
$\quad\quad\quad \downarrow \div 100$
3

This rule also works with decimals, for example $36 \div 10 = 3.6$, as shown below:

T   U   .   1/10
3   6   .   0
$\quad\quad\quad\quad \downarrow \div 10$
3   .   6

Similarly, $12.04 \div 100 = 0.1204$, as shown below (all digits have moved two places to the right):

T   U   .   1/10   1/100   1/1000   1/10,000
1   2   .   0   4
$\quad\quad\quad\quad\quad\quad\quad\quad \downarrow \div 100$
0   .   1   2   0   4

Activity 1.6

Try the following calculations:

1. $24 \div 10$ 3. $62.64 \div 10$ 5. $12 \div 1000$
2. $3.6 \div 100$ 4. $0.3 \div 100$

A quicker way of working

You may feel that you do not want or need to draw a place value chart every time you want to multiply or divide by 10, by 100 or by 1000. Many people find that, once they have grasped the concept, it is quicker and easier to concentrate on moving the decimal point rather than moving all of the digits within a chart. Using this quick method, you are imagining rather than drawing the place value columns. To demonstrate, here are the two methods of working out 0.6×10:

Using place value columns

U	.	1/10
0	.	6

$\downarrow \times 10$

6	.	0

$\leftarrow$ _____

Digit moves one place to the left. The answer is 6.

Moving the decimal point

0.6 $\times$ 10

0 6. 0

$\rightarrow$

Decimal point moves one place to the right. The answer is 6.

If there is no decimal point in the original number, insert it where it should be (for example, 12 becomes 12.0). This allows you to move it as required. This example shows 12 $\times$ 100 using the quick method of moving the decimal point:

12.0 $\times$ 100 becomes 1200.0

$\rightarrow$

The decimal point has moved two places to the right and the answer is 1200. Remember to fill any empty place value columns with zeros so that the digits are in the correct columns.

Similarly, 4.07 $\div$ 10 can be worked out using this quick method:

0.407

$\leftarrow$

The decimal point has moved one place to the left, and we have filled in the units column with a place holder zero. You can check these calculations using place value columns if you prefer.

Activity 1.7

Do the following calculations using whichever method feels most comfortable.

1. 2.4 $\div$ 100
2. 6.092 $\times$ 10
3. 0.3 $\div$ 1000
4. 0.3 $\times$ 1000

5. 92.1 $\div$ 100
6. 16 $\div$ 1000
7. 1.5 $\times$ 100

8. 0.0032 $\div$ 10
9. 8.408 $\times$ 100
10. 24,609.37 $\div$ 1000

SI units

The UK's healthcare system uses the International System of Units (*Système International d'Unités*) or SI units. This system was introduced in Britain in 1975. SI units are used when measuring weights, lengths, quantities of liquids and so on, to ensure that a unified standard is in use around the world and that everyone understands which units to use. SI units are used in almost every country for scientific and healthcare purposes. In this chapter, we will look at the units and quantities that you are most likely to encounter as a nurse. You will need SI units for measuring length (such as a patient's height), weight (of patients or tablets) and volume of liquids.

Length

The standard unit for measuring length is the metre, which is usually shortened to m (for example, twelve metres would be written as 12m). There are numerous related units that you need to be aware of:

- one kilometre (1km) = one thousand metres (1000m);
- one metre (1m) = one hundred centimetres (100cm);
- one centimetre (1cm) = ten millimetres (10mm);
- one metre (1m) = one thousand millimetres (1000mm).

Weight

Weights are measured using the gram (g). Again, there are numerous related units:

- one kilogram (1kg) = one thousand grams (1000g);
- one gram (1g) = one thousand milligrams (1000mg);
- one milligram (1mg) = one thousand micrograms (1000mcg).

Note: micrograms are sometimes written as μg, but this looks very similar to mg, which stands for milligrams (particularly when handwritten). Therefore, most people tend to write micrograms as mcg to avoid confusion, or you may even choose to write the word 'micrograms' out in full. It is recommended (*British National Formulary*, 2010) that micrograms and nanograms ('ng') should not be abbreviated.

Liquids

Liquids are measured using the litre (shortened to l or L):

- one litre (1L) = one thousand millilitres (1000ml).

Converting between units

As a nurse, you will need to know how to convert between related units, such as from millilitres to litres or from milligrams to micrograms. This is because prescriptions may, for example, specify a dose in milligrams, but the box of capsules on the shelf may describe the contents in micrograms. You will therefore need to know whether the box contains the correct strength of tablets, and you will do this by converting between related units.

Scenario

You have been asked to find 2000ml of saline solution, and the stock is all in one-litre pouches. How many do you need?

We know that one litre = 1000ml. So, we can multiply each side of this equation by two to reach our desired quantity of 2000ml (we must multiply both sides of the equation so that they are both still equal to each other):

$$1 \text{ litre} = 1000\text{ml}$$

↓ ×2   ↓ ×2

$$2 \text{ litres} = 2000\text{ml}$$

So, to find 2000ml of the saline solution, you will need two of the one-litre pouches.

However, it may not always be quite so straightforward. You might be asked to measure out 0.625 litres of the solution, but if your measuring scale is in millilitres, you will need to convert this amount from litres into millilitres in order to measure accurately. Again, we know that one litre = 1000ml. So, to get from 1 to 1000, we have multiplied by 1000. To measure out 0.625L, we need to convert this into millilitres by multiplying by 1000.

$$0.625 \times 1000 = 625$$
⟶

To multiply by 100, the decimal point has been moved three places to the right. Therefore, 0.625L = 625ml.

Activity 1.8

Using the information above and the techniques we looked at previously, work out the following conversions.

1. Convert 0.3 litres into millilitres.
2. Convert 36.7 litres into millilitres.
3. Convert 2.6L into ml.

Using the techniques shown earlier for multiplying and dividing by 10, by 100 and by 1000, you will be able to convert between any of the units mentioned. Table 1.1 sums up the calculations you will need.

The next activity tests how well you have grasped the topics we have looked at so far. You can use Table 1.1 to help you if you need it. However, be aware that you may not have a chart like this handy in your day-to-day activities.

Length		
Converting from	**Calculation**	**To**
km	× 1000	m
m	÷ 1000	km
m	× 100	cm
cm	÷ 100	m
cm	× 10	mm
mm	÷ 10	cm
m	× 1000	mm
mm	÷ 1000	m
Weight		
Converting from	**Calculation**	**To**
kg	× 1000	g
g	÷ 1000	kg
g	× 1000	mg
mg	÷ 1000	g
mg	× 1000	mcg
mcg	÷ 1000	mg
Volume of liquids		
Converting from	**Calculation**	**To**
L	× 1000	ml
ml	÷ 1000	L

Table 1.1: The calculations required when converting between SI units

Activity 1.9

Work out the following conversions.

1. Convert 25mm to cm.
2. Convert 3.2L to ml.

continued . . . •••

3. Convert 1.91m to cm.

4. Convert 86kg to g.

5. Convert 75mcg to mg.

6. Convert 0.2mg to mcg.

7. You have 250ml of water. How many litres is this?

8. A patient is prescribed 30mg of aripiprazole. How many grams is this?

9. You have a 500mg paracetamol tablet in front of you. How many mcg is this?

10. A patient requires 0.1mg of a drug per day. How many micrograms is this?

Addition

Case study

Remi, a registered nurse, had difficulties working out how many tablets of clozapine to adminster to her patient, Brenda. Brenda is prescribed clozapine 175mg at night. The pharmacy dispensed three boxes of Clozapine with 100mg, 25mg and 50mg tablets.

You will need to be able to add quantities together, including those that are given in different units, such as adding litres and millilitres. You might therefore need to convert between units before you can even begin adding, and it is vital that you check which units you are using before coming up with an answer, as dosage mistakes could have very serious consequences.

Adding whole numbers

When adding two or more numbers together, it is important to place each digit in the correct place value column, so that each number is worth the correct amount. You can then add the numbers in each column together, starting on the right with the units column and continuing column by column towards the left. For example, $32 + 16$ would be carried out like this:

$$
\begin{array}{r}
3 \quad 2 \\
+ \quad 1 \quad 6 \\
\hline
4 \quad 8 \\
\uparrow
\end{array}
$$

You have added $2 + 6$ in the units column (which equals 8) and then moved towards the left and added the $3 + 1$ in the tens column (which equals 4). The answer is therefore four tens and eight units, which is 48.

Sometimes, the answer you get in one column comes to more than ten, and you can only fit one digit in each column in your answer area. In the next example, you need to add 23 and 29 together. Adding the 3 and the 9 in the units column comes to 12. There are two digits in 12, so it cannot fit into the units column in your answer area. The 12 can be split into its constituent parts of 10 and 2. So, the 2 (units) is written in the units answer area, and the 1 (meaning 'one lot of ten') is 'carried over' into the tens column. It can then be added along with the other digits in the tens column, so that the answer contains the correct amount of tens:

$$
\begin{array}{r}
 2\quad 3 \\
 +\quad 2\quad 9 \\
 \hline
 5_1\quad 2 \\
 \uparrow
\end{array}
$$

The small digit 1 in the tens column has been carried over from the units column (2 + 2 = 4, add the 1 brings us to 5). You may be used to writing this digit in a different place in your working out – this is fine; you may write it wherever you are used to writing it, as long as you remember to add it on.

Adding with decimals

You may need to add decimal fractions to each other or to whole numbers. Again, it is very important that each digit is written in the correct place value column. The addition itself works in exactly the same way as shown above, starting from the column on the right and moving towards the left. You may need to insert some zeros as place holders in order to line up your place value columns and avoid mistakes. For example, to work out the sum 2.4 + 30.17:

These zeros have been added to make the sum easier to calculate.

$$
\begin{array}{r}
 0\quad 2\ .\ 4\quad 0 \\
 +\quad 3\quad 0\ .\ 1\quad 7 \\
 \hline
 3\quad 2\ .\ 5\quad 7
\end{array}
$$

As previously mentioned, you may need to convert between different units before you begin the sum itself, as you can only add quantities together that are given in the same unit. For example, a patient takes two paracetamol tablets, one weighing 0.5g and the other weighing 250mg. What is the total weight taken by the patient?

You cannot add 0.5g and 250mg together immediately, as grams and milligrams are very different in size. So you need to convert into the same units before you can begin adding. In this example, you have not been asked to give your answer in a particular unit, so it does not matter which units you choose to work with. Both answers are shown below.

By converting into grams

To convert 250mg into grams, we need to divide by 1000 (you can check this using the chart provided in Table 1.1):

$250 \div 1000 = 0.25$

We now need to add 0.25 to 0.5 (both numbers are now in grams):

```
      0  .  2   5
+     0  .  5   0
─────────────────
      0  .  7   5
```

The answer is 0.75g.

By converting into milligrams

To convert 0.5g into mg, we need to multiply by 1000:

$0.5 \times 1000 = 500$

So 0.5g = 500mg

We now need to add 250mg and 500mg, which gives us 750mg.

The answer is therefore 750mg.

Both answers are the same, because 750mg = 0.75g.

Be careful to give your answer in the correct units.

Activity 1.10

Work out the answers to the following.

1. $34.6 + 9.25$
2. You have 2.5 litres of water and add another 75ml to it. How much water do you now have? (Give your answer in litres.)
3. What is 2.5mg + 350mcg? (Give your answer in mcg.)

Subtraction

Otherwise known as 'taking away', you may need to subtract one quantity from another. As with addition, it is very important that each digit is written in the correct place value column. For example, $42 - 31$ would be written like this:

```
      4   2
−     3   1
─────────────
      1   1
```

Again, you need to start with the right-hand column and subtract the bottom digit from the top digit. In this example, you will therefore need to work out $2 - 1$ first, then $4 - 3$.

Sometimes, as in the next example of $732 - 514$, you may not be able to carry out the subtraction immediately, as you cannot take 4 away from 2. In this case, you need to 'borrow' a ten from the tens column as shown, and take 4 away from 12 instead:

$$
\begin{array}{r}
7 \quad 3^{2} \quad {}^{1}2 \\
- \quad 5 \quad 1 \quad 4 \\
\hline
2 \quad 1 \quad 8
\end{array}
$$

In the example above, we have 'borrowed' a ten from the tens column (the 3 has therefore become a 2 as there are now two tens not three). We have then moved this ten into the units column, making it hold twelve rather than two.

Note: you may be more used to using a different method of subtraction, and it is important that you use the method with which you feel most comfortable. The most common alternative method is called 'paying back', whereby the ten is not removed from the top row of the tens column but is 'paid back' to the bottom row instead. The answer will be exactly the same, and the above sum would look like this:

$$
\begin{array}{r}
7 \quad 3 \quad {}^{1}2 \\
- \quad 5 \quad {}^{2}1 \quad 4 \\
\hline
2 \quad 1 \quad 8
\end{array}
$$

Subtraction with decimals

As with addition, you subtract decimals in exactly the same way as you would subtract whole numbers. Make sure that your place value columns are lined up correctly, which may mean that you need to insert place holder zeros such as in the next example.

Work out the answer to $34 - 22.8$. You would set the sum out like this:

$$
\begin{array}{r}
3 \quad 4^{3} \quad . \quad {}^{1}0 \\
- \quad 2 \quad 2 \quad . \quad 8 \\
\hline
1 \quad 1 \quad . \quad 2
\end{array}
$$

The answer is therefore 11.2. Remember that you may need to convert between units before subtracting.

Activity 1.11

Try the following calculations, using whichever method you find most comfortable.

1. $53.9 - 14.21$
2. You have three litres of water and you use 25ml of it. How much is left, in millilitres?
3. At his or her first appointment, a patient weighs 82.5kg. By the second appointment, the patient weighs 76.25kg. How many grams has the patient lost?

Multiplication

Multiplication skills are essential when calculating drug doses. You will probably find it useful to practise your times tables (up to ten) before attempting this section, as long multiplication depends on them. You may be able to say your times tables in your head or out loud, or you might prefer to write them down. You might even feel more comfortable carrying a multiplication square around with you, like the one in Table 1.2, if you find your tables hard to remember. If you are struggling with them, think about what multiplication means and how you could fill in any gaps. For example, if you can remember that $6 \times 6 = 36$, but cannot recall 7×6, you can work out the answer by adding on another 6 to 36. Multiplication can be thought of as repeated addition: 3×2 can be thought of as 'three twos' or 'three lots of two'. As it involves small numbers, it can easily be worked out by repeatedly adding:

$$
\begin{array}{r}
2 \\
+ \quad 2 \\
2 \\
\hline
6
\end{array}
$$

Therefore, $3 \times 2 = 6$.

You can use this technique for helping you with your times tables or for working out smaller sums such as the following one.

You have two tablets, each weighing 25mg. What is the total weight of the tablets?

To answer this by repeated addition is easy:

$$
\begin{array}{r}
2 \quad 5 \\
+ \quad 2 \quad 5 \\
\hline
5 \quad 0
\end{array}
$$

The answer is 50g.

However, this method would be very difficult and time-consuming for larger quantities. Imagine you have 65 of those 25mg tablets – to answer this using repeated addition would take an incredibly long time and there would be a much greater chance of making a mistake. Using other multiplication techniques therefore makes such calculations far easier and less time-consuming.

Multiplying larger numbers by single-digit whole numbers

You have some tablets weighing 125mcg each. You weigh out nine of them – what will the total weight be?

This can be worked out by multiplying 125 by 9, and you would write it out like this:

$$
\begin{array}{r}
1 \quad 2 \quad 5 \\
\times \quad \underline{ 9}
\end{array}
$$

×	1	2	3	4	5	6	7	8	9	10
1	1	2	3	4	5	6	7	8	9	10
2	2	4	6	8	10	12	14	16	18	20
3	3	6	9	12	15	18	21	24	27	30
4	4	8	12	16	20	24	28	32	36	40
5	5	10	15	20	25	30	35	40	45	50
6	6	12	18	24	30	36	42	48	54	60
7	7	14	21	28	35	42	49	56	63	70
8	8	16	24	32	40	48	56	64	72	80
9	9	18	27	36	45	54	63	72	81	90
10	10	20	30	40	50	60	70	80	90	100

Table 1.2: Multiplication square

The 125 is made up of 5, 20 and 100, or five units, two tens and one hundred.

Starting with the units column, you then multiply each column in turn by nine. So, you work out 5×9, then 2×9, and then 1×9.

$$\begin{array}{cccc} & 1 & 2 & 5 \\ \times & & & 9 \\ \hline 1 & 1_2 & 2_4 & 5 \end{array}$$

You will have gone through the following stages.

- Work out 5×9. The answer is 45. As before, only one digit can fit in each column of the answer area, so the 5 is written in the answer area and the 4 (representing four tens or forty) is carried into the tens column to be added on to the answer there.
- Work out 2×9. The answer is 18. You then need to add the 4 you carried over, making a total of 22. Your answer for this column is 22 – as before, you need to carry the 2 which represents 20 into the next column, where it will be added to the answer for that column.
- Work out $1 \times 9 = 9$. You need to add the 2 you carried over, making a total of 11. As there are no more columns to multiply, you write 11 in the thousands and hundreds columns of the answer area.
- Your answer is 1125mcg. You have one thousand, one hundred (or eleven hundreds), one twenty and five units.
- Always remember which units you are using.

Multiplying decimals by single-digit whole numbers

Case study

Trish is a registered nurse who is administering medication to patients. She notices that Jane, a patient who suffers from schizophrenia, is prescribed olanzapine 7.5mg at night. However, she has run out of stock supply of 7.5mg tablets and what is left in stock is only 5mg, 2.5mg and 10mg olanzapine tablets. Because Trish cannot work out the arithmetic, she informs Jane that she has run out of the right tablets. She is unable to work out that she could give three tablets of 2.5mg or one tablet of 5mg and another of 2.5mg.

In the following example, you have nine tablets, each weighing 1.55mg. What is the total weight of all nine tablets?

Multiplying with decimals is the one area where it is advisable *not* to write the sum out in strict place value columns. Instead, you will probably find it easier to ignore the decimal point at first (we will come back to it later). So, to work out this sum, you would need to do this:

$$
\begin{array}{ccccc}
 & 1 & .5 & 5 & \\
\times & & & 9 & \\
\hline
1 & 3_4 & .9_4 & 5 & \text{mg}
\end{array}
$$

You will go through the following stages.

- Work out the sum as if the decimal point was not there at first.
- $5 \times 9 = 45$ (carry the 4 into the next column).
- $5 \times 9 = 45$, then add on the 4 you carried over, which gives you 49. Carry the 4 into the next column.
- $1 \times 9 = 9$, then add the 4 you carried over, $9 + 4 = 13$.
- You now have 1395. You need to replace the decimal point in the correct position. The trick to doing so is this: work out how many digits there are in the sum *after* the decimal point. In this example there are two (the two fives). You need the same number of digits after the decimal point in your answer, so replace the decimal point two places in from the right in your answer. In this case, this gives you 13.95.
- Your final answer is therefore 13.95mg.

This trick also includes any zeros in your answer, such as in the sum below – there are two digits after the decimal point in the question (3 and 4) so you need to have two digits after the decimal point in your answer (the 7 and 0 will be after the decimal point):

$$
\begin{array}{ccccc}
 & 2 & .3 & 4 & \\
\times & & & 5 & \\
\hline
1 & 1 & .7_2 & 0 &
\end{array}
$$

Try the questions in Activity 1.12 before moving on to the next section. Be careful to give your answer in the correct units.

Activity 1.12

Answer the following questions, using multiplication.

1. A patient is prescribed 250mg of carisoprodol, four times a day for three days. How much carisoprodol will the patient take in total, in grams?
2. A patient takes two 0.075g tablets of amoxicillin. How many milligrams does he or she take in total?

Long multiplication

Long multiplication is used when multiplying numbers of more than one digit by other numbers of more than one digit. There are several methods of doing this, and the most common is described here. If you are comfortable using a different method, you can continue using it when trying the activities in this section. For example, we will work out the answer to 73 × 24:

$$
\begin{array}{rr}
 & 7 \quad 3 \\
\times & 2 \quad 4 \\
\end{array}
$$

You cannot work this out immediately as the numbers are too big, so you need to break 24 into its constituent parts of 20 and 4. You can then multiply, in effect, 73 by 20 and then by 4. Adding these two answers together will give you the final answer to the original sum. It makes no difference in which order you do this (multiplying by the 20 first or by the 4), but as you may be used to working in only one of these ways, both are shown here.

Multiplying by the 4 first

$$
\begin{array}{rrrr}
 & & 7 & 3 \\
 & \times & 2 & 4 \\
\hline
 & 2 & 9_1 & 2 \\
+ & 1 \quad 4 & 6 & 0 \\
\hline
\end{array}
$$

You must insert this zero to show that you are multiplying by 20, not by 2. This zero moves all of the digits into their correct place value columns.

You will have gone through the following stages.

- 3 × 4 = 12 (carry the 1 into the next column).
- 7 × 4 = 28. Add the 1 you carried over, making 29.
- Move on to multiplying by 20 – insert a zero to show that you are actually multiplying by 20, not by 2. You then continue to multiply each column by 2.
- 3 × 2 = 6.
- 7 × 2 = 14.
- You now have two answers. You know that 73 × 4 = 292, and 73 × 20 = 1460. You need to add them together to find the total, which will give you the answer to 73 × 24.
- 292 + 1460 = 1752. Your answer is 1752.

Multiplying by the 20 first

$$
\begin{array}{r r r r}
 & & 7 & 3 \\
\times & & 2 & 4 \\
\hline
1 & 4 & 6 & 0 \\
+ & & 2 & 9_1 & 2 \\
\hline
1 & 7_1 & 5 & 2 \\
\end{array}
$$

As you can see, this gives exactly the same answer, as you have carried out the same calculation but in a very slightly different order. In this case, you have multiplied by the 20 first, so you need to put your zero place holder in the first answer row to show that you are multiplying by 20. As before, you then multiply 3×2, followed by 7×2. In the next stage, you multiply by the 4 (3×4 then 7×4). Again, adding the two answers you have come up with will give you the final answer ($1460 + 292 = 1752$).

Long multiplication with decimals

As shown before, it is often best to ignore the decimal point at first when multiplying with decimals. When you have reached an answer, replace the decimal point in the correct location to make sure that all digits are in the correct place value columns. For example, we need to find the answer to 28×1.5. Work out 28×15 first, then look to see how many digits appear after the decimal point in the original sum (in this sum, one digit appears after the decimal point). Place your decimal point so that the same number of digits appear after it (in this case, one):

$$
\begin{array}{r r r}
 & 2 & 8 \\
\times & 1 & .5 \\
\hline
2 & 8 & 0 \\
+ 1 & 4_4 & 0 \\
\hline
4_1 & 2 & .0 \\
\end{array}
$$

The answer is 42.0, which can then be shortened to 42. You can estimate whether your answer looks plausible – you are looking for one-and-a-half times 28, so you know that the answer is not going to be 420 or 4.2 (decimal point replaced in the wrong place).

Worked example

Find the answer to 9.34×6.1.

$$
\begin{array}{r r r r r}
 & 9 & .3 & 4 \\
\times & 6 & .1 \\
\hline
5 & 6_2 & 0_2 & 4 & 0 \\
+ & & 9 & 3 & 4 \\
\hline
5 & 6 & .9 & 7 & 4 \\
\end{array}
$$

In this sum, there are three digits after the decimal point (the three, the four and the one) so there must be three digits after the decimal point in the answer too. The answer is 56.974.

The questions in Activity 1.13 will give you the opportunity to practise using long multiplication. You can use a calculator to check your answers, but you need to be able to carry out these kinds of calculations without one.

Activity 1.13

Calculate the following, using whichever method of long multiplication you prefer.

1. 126 × 38
2. 96 × 2.3
3. 3.82 × 4.1
4. A patient takes one zopiclone 3.75mg tablet each day. How many milligrams will they take in a week?
5. Your patient is prescribed 1.75mg of alprazolam, three times a day. How much (in grams) will the patient take in a five-day period?

As mentioned earlier, you should use your judgement as to whether an answer looks right. You can get a rough idea of what the answer will be by estimating or rounding numbers. For example, if you need to work out 2.1 × 3.9, you could round it to 2 × 4 (2.1 is almost 2 and 3.9 is almost 4). You know that the answer therefore needs to be somewhere close to 8, and the correct answer is in fact 8.19. You can judge that your answer of 8.19 is likely to be correct as it is about right, whereas if you had come up with an answer of 81.9 you would be able to see that you had made a mistake.

Division

Division is often called 'sharing' as it is easiest to explain in terms of sharing one quantity with another. For example, you have a pizza that is cut into eight equal slices. You share it equally between four people – how many slices does each person receive? This one is easy, as you can visualise eight slices divided by four people. 8 ÷ 4 = 2. You can check your answer by multiplying the two slices each by the four people, that is 2 × 4 = 8. However, larger sums may be more difficult, and this is where various methods of short and long division will be useful. There are many different ways of dividing, and the most common is shown here (again, if you are comfortable with another method, you may use it to calculate the answers to the questions in this section).

Worked example

A patient is prescribed 75mg per day of their medicine. This needs to be spread between three equal doses at meal times. How large is each single dose?

To answer this question, you need to divide 75 by 3. You could write this out as 75 ÷ 3, but you may not be able to work it out in that way. You are probably familiar with division sums that look like this:

continued . . .

$$3 \overline{\smash{)}7\ 5}$$

This means 75 divided by 3, or how many threes are there in seventy-five. Working out this sum step by step gives us an answer of 25mg:

$$\overset{2\ \ 5}{3 \overline{\smash{)}7\ \ ^15}}$$

You will need to carry out the following stages.

*   Starting with the column on the left this time, you need to find out how many threes there are in seven.
*   The answer is two, so the digit 2 is placed above the 7 in the answer area. However, $3 \times 2 = 6$, so there is one left over. This needs to be 'carried over' into the next column, so the five becomes fifteen (you have actually been finding out how many threes there are in seventy, as the seven is in the tens column, so there is one ten left over. That is why the five becomes fifteen – you have carried a ten into the units column).
*   Now you need to find out how many threes there are in fifteen – there are five, so the digit 5 is written in the answer area.
*   Your answer to the sum is 25, as $75 \div 3 = 25$.
*   Remember you are working in milligrams, so each dose will weigh 25mg.

Dividing by two-digit numbers

This works in exactly the same way, even though it looks more complicated. For example, to find the answer to $144 \div 12$, you can do the following:

$$\overset{0\ \ 1\ \ 2}{12 \overline{\smash{)}1\ \ 4\ \ ^24}}$$

*   How many twelves are there in one? This cannot be done, so we place a zero in the answer area and carry the one over into the next column.
*   We now need to know how many twelves there are in fourteen. There is one, so we place a digit 1 in the answer area. There are also two left over, which we carry across into the next column.
*   How many twelves are there in twenty-four? There are exactly two, so we place a digit 2 in our answer area, giving us a final answer of 12.
*   Therefore, $144 \div 12 = 12$.

Remainders

Sometimes, the answer might not be as straightforward as in the examples above. One number might not divide exactly into the other, and you may have a quantity 'left over' – a remainder. As a nurse, you will always need to work out your answer accurately and give your answers as decimals, rather than something like 'four remainder one'. Bear in mind that 'four remainder one' is unlikely to equate to 4.1, so you will need to be able to work out answers to these kinds of questions accurately. The example below shows how you can work out the answer to 68 ÷ 8:

$$\begin{array}{r} 0 \;\; 8 \;\; . \;\; 5 \\ 8\,\overline{\smash{)}6 \;\; 8 \;\; . \;\; {}^4 0} \end{array}$$

You need to go through the following stages.

- How many eights in six? You cannot do this, so place a zero in the answer area.
- How many eights in sixty-eight? $8 \times 8 = 64$, so there are eight with four left over. Place the eight in the answer area and carry the four over to the next column.

As there is no 'next column' yet, you need to insert the decimal point where it would be (68.0) and carry the four over so that the next column becomes 40. You are now looking for how many eights there are in forty.

There are five eights in forty, with nothing left over. Remember to place the decimal point in the answer area, directly about the decimal point in the sum itself. Your answer is 8.5 (note that eight remainder four did not equate to eight point four).

Dividing whole numbers into decimal numbers

This works in exactly the same way as the example above. Imagine you need to divide 12.5mg of a medicine into four equal doses. You could work out the sum like this:

$$\begin{array}{r} 0 \;\; 3 \;\; . \;\; 1 \;\; 2 \;\; 5 \\ 4\,\overline{\smash{)}1 \;\; 2 \;\; . \;\; 5 \;\; {}^1 0 \;\; {}^2 0} \end{array}$$

- How many fours are there in twelve? There are three.
- How many fours are there in five? There is one, with one left over. You therefore need to carry the one into the next column and add another zero to the sum (12.5 becomes 12.50).
- You can then find out how many fours there are in ten. There are two, with two left over, so repeat the process of adding another zero.
- You are now looking for the number of fours in twenty. There are exactly five.
- Your answer is 3.125mg per dose.

The next activity gives you the opportunity to practise the kinds of division questions we have looked at so far.

Activity 1.14

Try the following calculations.

1. 186 ÷ 6
2. 169 ÷ 13
3. 103.5 ÷ 6
4. 99.2 ÷ 8
5. 21.35 ÷ 7

Dividing by a decimal

We have already looked at dividing *into* a decimal number. However, you may need to divide *by* a decimal number. If you have a pile of tablets with a total weight of 15g, and you know that each tablet weighs 2.5g, how can you use written division to find out how many tablets are in the pile? You need to calculate $15 \div 2.5$:

$$2.5 \overline{\smash{\big)}\ 1\ \ 5}$$

However, finding out how many two-point-fives there are in another number is quite tricky. Ideally, we want to be dividing by a whole number, so we want to get rid of the decimal point. We cannot just remove it, but we can multiply each side of the sum by ten in order to get rid of the decimal point without changing the proportion of the sum. For example, $4 \div 2$ and $40 \div 20$ will give you exactly the same answer (two) – each 'side' of the sum has been multiplied by ten so the proportion of the sum remains the same. If we had only multiplied one side of the sum by ten but not the other, we would have ended up with either $40 \div 2$ (which equals 20) or $2 \div 40$ (which equals 0.05). These are both rather different answers. It is therefore vital that we multiply both sides of the sum when 'getting rid of' a decimal point in this way.

Therefore, our original sum of $15 \div 2.5$ now becomes $150 \div 25$. In this example, there are six tablets in the pile:

$$25 \overline{\smash{\big)}\ \overset{0\ \ \ 0\ \ \ 6}{1\ \ \ 5\ \ \ 0}}$$

Activity 1.15

Answer the following questions using written methods of division.

1. $75 \div 1.2$
2. A pack of tablets weighs 90mg, excluding the packaging. Each individual tablet weighs 1.5mg. How many tablets are in the pack?
3. A box containing capsules weighs 250g in its entirety. The box itself weighs 30g, and each capsule weighs 0.5g. How many capsules are in the box?

In the chapter so far, we have looked at addition, subtraction, multiplication and division (the 'four rules of number'). We have also looked at decimals and how to calculate with them, and at units of measure along with how to convert between them. There are a few more topics that you will need to be familiar with, and these are discussed below.

Ratio

Simply put, a ratio is the relationship between two quantities. Imagine you are making some orange squash. You use a cordial-to-water ratio of 1:4 (one to four). This means that, for every one cup of cordial you use, you will need four cups of water. Similarly, for every 100ml of cordial used, there will be 400ml of water. If you use 250ml of cordial, you will need 1000ml (or one litre) of water, and the entire drink will measure 1.25 litres (1250ml).

Worked example

At a party, the ratio of men to women is 3:2. If there are 24 men at the party, how many women are there?

$$
\begin{array}{ccc}
\text{Men} & : & \text{Women} \\
3 & : & 2 \\
\times 8 \downarrow & & \downarrow \times 8 \\
24 & : & 16
\end{array}
$$

We have multiplied the three by eight to get 24, so we must therefore multiply the two by eight as well – this gives us an answer of 16 women (and a total number of guests of 24 + 16 = 40).

You may come across ratios when diluting medicines or finding the correct strength drug. Many drugs are available in solutions of different strengths, and it is very important that you choose the correct one. Imagine the orange squash again. A cordial-to-water ratio of 1:4 means that there are five 'parts' to the mixture (one cup of cordial plus four cups of water equals five cups of liquid in total). Therefore, the cordial represents one out of the five parts, or 1/5, and may be referred to as a '1 in 5' solution (the cordial is one of the five parts). If we made our squash in a 1:10 ratio, it would be much weaker or less concentrated, as there would be eleven 'parts' and the cordial only represents one of them. This would be 1/11 or a '1 in 11' solution.

The same applies to medicines you will encounter as a nurse. A solution with a concentrate to water ratio of 1:100 is much stronger than a solution whose concentrate to water ratio is 1:10,000. As ever, you must be very careful with your units to ensure that you are finding the correct dose and have not confused your litres and millilitres.

You will probably see strengths of solutions written in the format mg/ml, or milligrams per millilitre. This refers to the amount of milligrams of active ingredient (drug) found in one millilitre of the solution. A solution with a strength of 5mg/ml has 5mg of the active ingredient in every millilitre of liquid. Therefore, ten millilitres of the solution will provide fifty milligrams of the drug itself. We will return to calculations using quantities like this shortly.

Percentages

'Per cent' means 'out of one hundred', and refers to how much of something you have. For example, fifty-five **per cent** (55%) means fifty-five out of every hundred. It could also be written as a **fraction** (55/100), or as a decimal (0.55, meaning we have fifty-five hundredths). To find

55 per cent of something, you can multiply it by 0.55. To find 43 per cent, multiply by 0.43 and so on. You change the percentage into a decimal (how many hundredths do you have?) and multiply your original number by this decimal. For example, to find 25 per cent of 40, change the 25 per cent into a decimal (0.25) and multiply the original number by this. $0.25 \times 40 = 10$, so 25 per cent of 40 is 10.

As with ratios, you will probably see percentages used to describe the strengths of solutions. Looking at the orange squash example again, if the drink made is up of cordial and water, and cordial represents 10 per cent of the squash, water must make up 90 per cent ($10\% + 90\% = 100\%$). Similarly, if dithranol ointment has a strength of 2 per cent, it means that 2g out of every 100g is the active ingredient. A 200g tube of ointment will contain 4g of active ingredient, and so on.

Drug strengths or concentrations may be expressed as:

- w/v (weight in volume) used when solids are dissolved in water to make solutions;
- w/w (weight in weight) when solids are dissolved in other solids, such as creams or ointments);
- v/v (volume in volume) when liquids are mixed into other liquids).

It is important to remember the following when calculating drug concentrations:

- one litre of water weighs one kilogram;
- one millilitre of water weighs one gram.

These weights are taken to be accurate for drug calculation purposes. So, a 20 per cent w/v solution means that 20g of a drug has been dissolved in every 100ml of water ($20\% = 20$ out of 100, so if there is 20g of a drug dissolved, it must be in 100ml of water as $1g = 1ml$).

Activity 1.16

Answer the following questions, which are about ratio and percentages.

1. What weight, in grams, of glucose is dissolved in two litres of a solution with a strength of 10 per cent w/v?
2. How many grams of active ingredient are dissolved in 15ml of 5 per cent w/v solution?
3. How many grams of hydrocortisone are there in 200g of a cream with a strength of 1 per cent w/w?
4. Another batch of hydrocortisone cream is mixed with base ingredients to a ratio of 1:49. You have 100g of the cream. How many grams are of the active ingredient?
5. Which cream is stronger (contains more active ingredient), the cream in question 3 or the cream in question 4?

If you have found any of the questions so far difficult, it may help to read over the relevant sections of this chapter before moving on.

Drug calculation formulae

You have already carried out many of the common calculations you will need as a nurse. There are some formulae with which you need to familiarise yourself, as they will be very useful to you in your career. However, as explained at the very beginning of this chapter, you cannot rely on trying to follow a formula simply by using a calculator. You need to understand the stages you are going through, and must be able to spot and correct any mistakes you make. This chapter so far has looked at the numeracy skills you will need and how to apply these to real situations. This section looks at the formulae that will help you, and how to use them effectively using the skills you have been developing.

How many tablets?

The formula for working out how many tablets or capsules you will need is as follows:

$$\frac{\text{Amount prescribed}}{\text{Amount available in each tablet}} = \text{number of tablets you need}$$

Worked example

A patient is prescribed 45mg of olanzapine per day, to be taken in one dose. The available tablets contain 15mg each. How many tablets does the patient need to take?

$$\frac{45}{15} = 3$$

(45/15 means the same as $45 \div 15$, or how many fifteens there are in forty-five.) You can check this by working out $3 \times 15 = 45$.

How many tablets by body weight?

Sometimes you will need to calculate dosage according to the body weight of the patient. This is more common in children's nursing. This will be given in, say, milligrams per kilogram of body weight (mg/kg). The formula to help you is:

Body weight (kg) $\times$ dose per kg = dose required

Worked example

A patient who weighs 80kg is prescribed a dose of 10mg/kg. How much does the patient require?

$80 \times 10 = 800\text{mg}$

How much liquid?

The formula for calculating how much of a liquid you need is:

$$\frac{\text{Amount prescribed}}{\text{Amount available (strength)}} \times \text{volume the drug is in} = \text{required volume}$$

In other words:

$$\frac{\text{How much you need}}{\text{What strength you have}} \times \text{volume it's in} = \text{volume to give to patient}$$

Worked example

You need to get a dose of a drug ready for a patient. The drug is available in 250mg in 10ml (250mg of the active ingredient has been dissolved into every 10ml of the liquid), and you need 100mg of it. What volume of the solution is needed?

$$\frac{100}{250} \times 10 =$$

Dividing first

$$250\,\overline{\smash)\begin{array}{c}0\ \ 0\ \ 0\ \ .\ \ 4 \\ 1\ \ 0\ \ 0\ \ .\ \ 0\end{array}}$$

$0.4 \times 10 = 4$ml

Multiplying first

$100 \times 10 = 1000$

$1000 \div 250$

$$= 250\,\overline{\smash)\begin{array}{c}0\ \ 0\ \ 0\ \ .\ \ 4 \\ 1\ \ 0\ \ 0\ \ .\ \ 0\end{array}}$$

$= 4$ml

There are two ways to continue from this point. You can either divide first, or multiply first. As you can see from the example given, for this formula it does not matter which part of the sum you do first – the answer is the same. You can therefore either multiply or divide first, depending on which you find easier or on which numbers you have in your equation. We can demonstrate that this is the case for this formula by using simple numbers:

$$\frac{4}{2} \times 3 =$$

Dividing first

$4 \div 2 = 2$

$2 \times 3 = 6$

Multiplying first

$4 \times 3 = 12$

$12 \div 2 = 6$

Activity 1.17

The following questions are designed to test your ability to answer realistic problems that you may face in your job, using the techniques, skills and formulae discussed throughout this chapter.

1. Some tablets weigh 62.5mcg each. Your patient requires 0.25mg of the drug in total. How many tablets will you give the patient?
2. A patient requires 10mg of olanzapine by intramuscular injection. You have vials of olanzapine available which each contain 10mg and require 2.1ml of water to be added to them in order to reconstitute the drug ready for injection. The patient will be given an identical dose later in the day. How many ml of water will you use throughout the entire day?
3. Your patient needs 14mg of metoclopramide. The solution you have available contains 10mg in 2ml. How many ml will you need to give the patient, so that they receive the correct amount of the drug?
4. A patient is prescribed an antipsychotic injection. The required dose is 20mg. The stock you have contains 50mg in 2ml. How much do you need to administer?
5. You need to prepare 0.25g of sulphasalazine. The available medicine is 500mg in 5ml. How much do you give the patient?
6. Your patient is prescribed a weight-dependent drug at a dose of 2mg/kg every eight hours. The patient weighs 85kg. How much in mg will they receive in a 24- hour period?
7. Chlorpromazine is prescribed as a dose of 20mg every 6 hours. Your ampoules contain 10mg in one ml. How much (in ml) will be given in 24 hours?
8. A patient is prescribed 40mg of loxapine, divided between two doses a day. You only have 10mg tablets available at the moment. How many tablets per day would you need to give the patient?

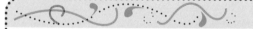

Chapter summary

In this chapter, we have looked at the numeracy skills you will need as a nurse, and at the kinds of calculations you will need to be able to do. We looked at place value, and how the position of each digit is vital in determining the value of a number. Using this knowledge, we then discussed how to multiply and divide by 10, by 100 and by 1000, before applying this to converting between SI units of measure. You have practised addition, subtraction, multiplication and division, with whole numbers and decimals. There was also information about ratio and percentages, and how these might be relevant to nursing. Finally, we studied the drug calculation formulae that will help you as a mental health nurse, and used all of the techniques covered within the chapter to answer realistic questions using these formulae.

Activities: answers

Activity 1.2 (page 8)
1. 2
2. Twenty-four million, eighty-six thousand and seventy-nine. Written out with place value columns, this would be:

TM	M	HTh	TTh	Th	H	T	U
2	4	0	8	6	0	7	9

TM means 'tens of millions'.
M means 'millions'.
HTh means 'hundreds of thousands' and so on.
3. 3,200,650
4. The millions column (1,000,000).
5. The tens of thousands column (10,000).

Activity 1.3 (page 9)
1.

T	U	.	1/10	1/100
£1	4	.	0	3

2. It is in the 'hundredths' column, and represents six hundredths.
3. The thousandths column.
4. 1.2 is bigger, as it represents one whole number and two tenths. 1.09 represents one whole number and nine hundredths (hundredths are smaller than tenths). It may help you to visualise this if you think of the amounts as money, i.e. £1.20 and £1.09.

Activity 1.4 (page 10)
1. 3,000
2. 2,900
3. 860
4. 346,200
5. 70,000

Activity 1.5 (page 10)
1. 1250
2. 3490.4
3. 66,200

Activity 1.6 (page 11)
1. 2.4
2. 0.036
3. 6.264
4. 0.003
5. 0.012

Activity 1.7 (page 12)
1. 0.024
2. 60.92
3. 0.0003
4. 300
5. 0.921
6. 0.016
7. 150
8. 0.00032
9. 840.8
10. 24.60937

Activity 1.8 (page 14)
1. 300ml
2. 36,700ml
3. 2600ml

Activity 1.9 (pages 15–16)
1. 2.5cm
2. 3200ml
3. 191cm
4. 86,000g
5. 0.075mg
6. 200mcg
7. 0.25L
8. 0.03g
9. 500,000mcg
10. 100mcg

Activity 1.10 (page 18)
1. 43.85
2. 75ml = 0.075L

$$
\begin{array}{ccccc}
  & 2 & . & 5 & & \\
+ & 0 & . & 0 & 7 & 5 \\
\hline
  & 2 & . & 5 & 7 & 5 \\
\end{array}
$$

The answer is 2.575 litres.

3. 2.5mg = 2500mcg

$$
\begin{array}{cccc}
  & 2 & 5 & 0 & 0 \\
+ & & 3 & 5 & 0 \\
\hline
  & 2 & 8 & 5 & 0 \\
\end{array}
$$

The answer is 2850mcg.

Activity 1.11 (page 19)
1.

$$
\begin{array}{ccccc}
  & {}^45 & {}^13 & . & {}^89 & {}^10 \\
- & 1 & 4 & . & 2 & 1 \\
\hline
  & 3 & 9 & . & 6 & 9 \\
\end{array}
$$

The answer is 39.69

2. 3 litres = 3000ml
$3000 - 25 = 2975$

The answer is 2975ml.

3. $82.50 - 76.25 = 06.25$
6.25kg = 6250g

The answer is 6250g.

Activity 1.12 (page 23)
1. 250mg × 4 times a day = 1000mg
1000mg × 3 days = 3000mg
3000mg = 3g total dose

The answer is 3g.

2. You can work this out in two ways:
   a) By converting g to mg first:
      0.075g = 75mg
      $75 \times 2 = 150$
      Total = 150mg.
   b) By multiplying first:
      $0.075 \times 2 = 0.150$
      This is 0.15g.
      Convert to mg: 0.15g = 150mg.

Activity 1.13 (page 25)
1. 4788
2. 220.8
3. 15.662
4. 26.25mg
5. 0.02625g

Activity 1.14 (page 27)

1. 31
2. 13
3. 17.25
4. 12.4
5. 3.05

The working out is shown here.

(a)
```
      0  3   1
   6 | 1  8   6
```

(b)
```
       0  1   3
   13 | 1  6  ³9
```

(c)
```
      0  1   7  .  2   5
   6 | 1  0  ⁴3  . ¹5  ³0
```

(d)
```
      1   2  .  4
   8 | 9  ¹9  . ³2
```

(e)
```
      0  3  .  0  5
   7 | 2  1  .  3  5
```

Activity 1.15 (page 28)

1. 62.5
2. 60 tablets
3. 440 capsules

The working out is shown here.

(a)
```
   1.2 | 7  5
```
```
        0  6   2  .  5
   12 | 7  5  ³0  . ⁶0
```

(b)
```
   1.5 | 9  0
```
```
        0  6  0
   15 | 9  0  0
```

(c)

250g	−	30g	=	220g
(total weight	−	weight of box	=	weight of capsules)

$220 \div 0.5 = 440$

Activity 1.16 (page 30)

1. 2 litres = 2000ml. Divide by 10 to find 10% = 200ml. We know that 1ml = 1g, so there are 200g of glucose. The answer is 200g.
2. 15ml = 15g. We need 5 per cent of this. We know that 5% = 5/100 or five hundredths (0.05), so if we multiply 15 by 0.05 we will find 5% of 15. 15 × 0.05 = 0.75. The answer is 0.75g.
3. 1 per cent of 200 = 2g.
4. 1:49 ratio means there are 50 parts. 50 × 2 = 100g. This means we must multiply both sides of the ratio by 2, giving us a ratio of 2:98. 2g + 98g = 100g. Therefore we have 2g active ingredient. The answer is 2g.

5. The cream in question 4 is stronger, as there are 2g of active ingredient in every 100g (the other cream has 2g active in every 200g, or 1g active in every 100g).

Activity 1.17 (page 33)

1. 62.5mcg = 0.0625mg
   $0.0625 \times 4 = 0.25$mg
   So, we need 4 tablets.

2. 2.1ml $\times$ 2 = 4.2ml of water in total (there are 2 doses, each requiring 2.1ml of water).

3. $\frac{14}{10} \times 2 = 1.4 \times 2 = 2.8$ml

   The answer is 2.8ml.

4. $\frac{20}{50} \times 2 = 0.8$ml

   The answer is 0.8ml.

5. 0.25 (grams) $\times$ 1000 = 250mg

   $\frac{250}{500} \times 5 = 2.5$ml

   The answer is 2.5ml.

6. $85 \times 2 = 170$mg every 8 hours.
   $24 \div 8 = 3$, so we need 3 doses.
   3×170mg = 510mg in 24 hours.

   The answer is 510mg.

7. $\frac{20}{10} \times 1 = 2$ml each dose
   $24 \div 6 = 4$ doses in total.
   2ml $\times$ 4 = 8ml in 24 hours.

   The answer is 8ml.

8. 40mg divided between 2 doses means 20mg per dose ($40 \div 2 = 20$).
   Each tablet weighs 10mg, so each dose requires 2 tablets.
   2 doses per day means 2 tablets $\times$ 2 doses = 4 tablets.

   The answer is 4 tablets in total.

Further reading

Haighton, J, Phillips, B, Thomas, V and Holder, D (2004) *Math: The basic skills* (curriculum edition). Cheltenham: Nelson Thornes.

An excellent resource for practising your numeracy skills.

Starkings, S and Krause, L (2010) *Passing Drugs Calculations Tests for Nursing Students*. Exeter: Learning Matters.

This up-to-date text is written specifically for nursing students and covers drugs calculations in detail.

Useful websites

www.mathcentre.ac.uk

This website has useful sections about drug calculations and general numeracy skills.

Chapter 2
Legal and ethical aspects of medicines management in mental health

Chapter aims

By the end of this chapter, you should be familiar with:

- accountability as a concept and four different areas of accountability;
- legislation that impacts on medicines management, along with types of prescribers;

- patient group directions (PGDs);
- ethical considerations in treatment, including coercion.

Introduction: a little history

Before 1919 there was no register of nurses, and no national regulation or standards for nurse training. At that time nurse training was normally for one year, and the general view was that most of what was essential could be learnt in that short time; but it became clear that a longer period of training for nurses was necessary to produce a 'professional' nurse.

The Nurses Registration Act of 1919 ended many years of conflict within the profession and set standards for training, examination and registration; this introduced to nursing the concept of legal accountability, which serves to protect the public from malpractice. This chapter will outline the concept of accountability in nursing before discussing specific legislation. It will then discuss the Human Rights, Mental Capacity and Mental Health Acts before reviewing legislation that deals directly with medicines, such as the Medicines Act, Drugs Misuse Act and the Nurse Prescribing Act. In addition, this chapter will briefly discuss ethical issues that arise when patients are given compulsory treatment.

Accountability

In common language, accountability may simply mean responsibility to someone or for some activity. In ethics and governance, the term is often used synonymously with concepts such as responsibility, answerability, blameworthiness and liability. However, Swansburg and Swansburg (2002) p364 defined accountability as:

> *The fulfilment of a formal obligation to disclose to referent others the purposes, principles, procedure, relationship, results, income, and expenditure for which one has authority.*

The Nursing and Midwifery Council (2008) states that:

> *You are personally accountable for your action and omission in your practice to a higher authority with whom you have a legal relationship.*

Although the word accountability has been used interchangeably with responsibility, it is important to make a clear distinction. Responsibility means having control or authority over someone or something. You can choose to take responsibility but you have no power to decide who you should be accountable to.

Scenario

Tom, a registered nurse who had no prescribing powers, altered his patient Tina's medicine chart for diazepam from 15mg to 20mg a day without consulting the prescriber. He administered this dose to the patient for a

continued . . .

> *week before it was brought to the attention of his manager. Tom argued that he knew Tina very well and she was always prescribed 20mg a day; and he believed it was perfectly within his rights to 'correct' the dose. He was disciplined by his employer and dismissed from his post.*

In the above scenario, Tom was responsible for adjusting the patient's dose and it was his choice to do so. However, he was accountable to his employers for his action and it was his employers, not him, who decided to terminate his employment.

The purpose of accountability

The principle of holding you accountable as a nurse is to ensure that the public and your patients are not harmed by your acts and omissions, and to provide redress to those who have been harmed. To achieve this, accountability has the following aims.

- The public must be protected from your acts or omissions that might cause harm. You can be called to account for your conduct and competence if it is thought you have fallen below the standards required of you.
- You must be held to account in order to protect the public and patients by discouraging you from acting in a way that would be considered as misconduct or unlawful. As a registered nurse you must act at all times in a manner worthy of a nurse at work, both in public and in private.
- To make you accountable to a range of higher authorities, the law regulates your behaviour. The regulatory framework makes it clear what standards of conduct and competence you are required to comply with as a registered nurse.

As a nurse you can be called to account and asked to justify your actions. Your case can be heard in public with a view to reassuring patients that only the highest standards of nursing will be tolerated. The public scrutiny of a nurse's conduct allows other members of the profession to learn from the mistakes and misconduct of others (Griffith and Tengnah, 2008).

Scenario

A registered nurse was struck off the professional register in 2010 after he was found sleeping on duty and had failed to administer medication to patients in a nursing home. He had initially denied the charges and later admitted to the offence after other employees had testified he had been caught sleeping on three separate occasions within two months. The committee found him unworthy of being a registered nurse.

Because you have a formal obligation to answer for your actions to a number of higher authorities, you have to justify your actions to these authorities and, if you fail to do so, sanctions can be applied against you. For example, in your training, your university or the NHS Trust can take disciplinary action against you which, in extreme cases, can result in your dismissal. In this regard, in general, you are accountable to:

- your patient;
- your professional body;
- society;
- your employer.

Accountability to your patient

As a nurse you are accountable to the patient who is under your care and, for this reason, civil law allows the patient to seek redress if they believe they have suffered harm due to your actions. Over the years, the NHS has been paying out increasingly large sums of money – over half a billion pounds a year – because of the clinical negligence of staff. A fundamental ethic of healthcare is that you should do your patients no harm. Where harm occurs as a result of your negligence, patients can seek compensation from you and your employers through the courts. The nurse–patient relationship gives rise to a duty of care and, therefore, you have a duty both to care and not to be careless.

Quite often nurses have argued that they are accountable to themselves for their practice. Although it is accepted that a nurse who harms a patient through their omissions will feel remorse, if the definition of accountability is taken into account, we see that nurses cannot impose sanctions on themselves.

Accountability to your professional body

As a registered nurse you are accountable to your professional body in accordance with the Nurses, Midwives and Health Visitors Act 1997. This legislation's aim is to protect the public by establishing standards for education, training and conduct. The basis of the NMC's role is the nursing register on which those who intend to practise as nurses are placed. A detailed description of the role of the NMC is beyond the scope of this book, so you are advised to consult a more appropriate textbook in this regard.

Accountability to society

As a nurse you are subject to the laws of the country you work in, like everyone else. If you are accused of committing a crime at work or outside work, you will be called to account under the laws of the country in which you reside. This can have a bearing on your ability to practise as a nurse, as demonstrated by the scenario below.

Scenario

Bridget was a registered nurse working in prison but was later arrested and convicted of supplying Class A drugs to a prison inmate. She was sentenced to three years and was subsequently removed from the professional register.

Accountability to your employer

As a nurse you are accountable to your employing organisation through the terms and conditions of your employment contract. An employer is vicariously liable for the actions of its employees. For example, if a nurse commits a civil wrong, the employer is responsible for the nurse's action. The following scenario gives an example of what this means in practice.

Scenario

Hamid is a patient on phenobarbitone who was found unconscious after a nurse, Shelley, gave him three times the dose prescribed. Hamid had to be admitted to a hospital intensive care ward and recovered fully four days later. The mistake occurred because Shelley did not follow correct procedures for administration of medicines. Although Hamid survived, his family persuaded him to take legal action through the courts and he won a substantial settlement from the hospital. In turn, Shelley was disciplined and was sent for retraining in medicines management.

In the scenario above, we see that Hamid came to some harm because of Shelley's carelessness. However, it was the hospital that was sued and paid compensation to the patient, not the nurse. The hospital is vicariously liable. Vicarious liability is a legal term that holds one person liable for the actions of another when engaged in some form of joint or collective venture. Both the hospital and the nurse can be said to be engaged in a collective venture, but the hospital has vicarious liability.

As previously mentioned, accountability is informed by various pieces of legislation, and these will be discussed next.

Human Rights Act 1998

Rights can be defined as claims or entitlements that deserve respect. After the Second World War, nations around the world were determined to take steps to guarantee the protection of human rights in international and national law. The first concrete manifestation of this was the American Declaration of the Rights and Duties of Man in 1948. This was followed by the Universal Declaration of Human Rights drawn up by the United Nations. These documents concentrated on protecting civil and political rights, such as freedom of expression, freedom of religion and freedom of association.

In the UK, human rights are enshrined in the Human Rights Act 1998, which was based on the European Convention on Human Rights (ECHR).

All public authorities have a legal duty to act compatibly with the ECHR (and hence the Human Rights Act). The National Health Service (NHS) is a public authority and therefore comes under the Act. Domestic courts are obliged to interpret all laws consistently with the Act. In mental health, courts and mental health tribunals are obliged to interpret the Mental Health Act 1983 consistently with the Human Rights Act 1998. The Human Rights Act thus has the effect of bringing human rights to the centre of both the legal and the health systems.

The ECHR is divided into 'articles', which set out the rights that are protected by the Convention. For the purpose of medicines management in mental health, only articles 2, 3 and 8 are relevant and it is these that we will discuss next.

Article 2

This article states that *Everyone's right to life shall be protected by law. No one shall be deprived of his life intentionally save in the execution of a sentence of a court following his conviction of a crime for which this penalty is provided by law.*

The article imposes on the state the obligation to protect the lives of its citizens and this responsibility extends to the healthcare system. Before you go further, please complete Activity 2.1.

Activity 2.1   *Reflection*

You are working on a ward where a patient, detained under section 3 of the Mental Health Act 1983, has attacked a fellow patient, causing serious harm. The aggressor was physically restrained and placed in seclusion to allow time for him to 'cool down'. He was then given an injection of olanzapine 10mg and a concomitant (augmenting) dose of lorazepam 2mg. Two hours after the administration of the injection, the patient went to sleep (at 1900 hours). Although the hospital policy stipulated clearly that a patient who is administered intramuscular olanzapine must have vital signs monitored regularly, this was not done for fear of waking the patient, and also there was insufficient staff on duty to cope with any potential acts of violence during that night.

Five hours later, staff found the patient unconscious and immediately sent him to the local general hospital where he was taken to the intensive care unit. After a period in hospital, he recovered fully but sued the hospital for breaching his rights under the Human Rights Act 1998.

- Is the hospital in breach of article 2 of the Human Rights Act?

An outline answer is provided at the end of the chapter.

The most obvious example of the application of article 2 is in cases where a member of staff deliberately kills a patient, as in the Harold Shipman cases (see 'Useful websites'), but article 2 extends beyond that as exemplified by a test case (*Stewart* v. *United Kingdom* [1984]). Moreover, it is not necessary for the victim to die to be in breach of article 2. It is sufficient to put the person at 'material risk', as the above scenario demonstrates. Clearly, it was the responsibility of the nursing staff to observe the patient's vital signs regularly after administering an intramuscular injection of olanzapine and lorazepam, but this was not done. The staff therefore placed the patient at material risk by their action, therefore breaching article 2.

Article 2 further stipulates that, where there is a threat to the life of someone in state custody (in this case the hospital), there is a heightened responsibility to provide care and protection. In the UK, this was brought about by a test case of *Osman* v. *United Kingdom* [2000]. After the death of a family member, a family sued the police for failing to protect them adequately. The judge in the case commented that, where the authorities know of a 'real and immediate threat' to a person's life, there is an obligation to take preventive operational measures to protect that person.

As a mental health nurse, you are likely to work in custodial environments such as a prison, secure hospital or immigration detention centre. Occasionally, you will be asked to comment on patient risks to themselves and to others. Therefore, you have a duty not only to the individual patient but also to the wider secure community of detained people, and your understanding of article 2 of the ECHR is important in formulating a decision.

Article 3

Article 3 of the European Convention on Human Rights is the only absolute right and it states: *No one shall be subjected to torture or to inhuman or degrading treatment or punishment.* In the UK, the courts have defined degrading treatment as:

> *Where treatment humiliates or debases an individual, showing lack of respect for, or diminishing, his or her human dignity, or arouses feelings of fear, anguish or inferiority capable of breaking an individual's moral and physical resistance, it may be characterised as degrading and also fall within the prohibition of Article 3. The suffering that naturally flows from naturally occurring illness, physical or mental, may be covered by Article 3, where it is, or risks being, exacerbated by treatment, whether flowing from conditions of detention, expulsion or other measures, for which the authorities can be held responsible.*
> (*Pretty* v. *United Kingdom* [2002])

Activity 2.2   *Reflection*

Having read the definition of degrading treatment, can you list situations in mental health nursing that could be described as degrading treatment, therefore breaching article 3 of the ECHR?

Read on for a discussion of this topic.

Although article 3 is an absolute right that is stated in very simple terms, the problem is that it can be interpreted in a variety of ways. Whether a particular deed is considered inhuman or degrading treatment will depend on a number of factors and the unique circumstances of each case. In mental health practice, article 3 is most likely to be relevant to complaints arising from the conditions of detention, seclusion, forced medication, control and restraint.

Case study

In Herczegfalvy v. Austria *[1992], Mr Herczegfalvy was a Hungarian citizen living in Austria who had served two prison sentences in succession for assaulting his wife, public officials and customers of his television repair business. In prison, he carried on assaulting fellow prisoners and prison staff. After an assessment, he was deemed to be suffering from a paranoid psychotic disorder and not responsible for his actions and was therefore sent to a psychiatric hospital.*

Following an assessment in the psychiatric hospital he was returned to prison, but he protested against his detention by staging a hunger strike and collapsed four weeks later needing intensive medical care. He was sent to a general hospital for treatment.

On his return to the psychiatric hospital, he was still on hunger strike but was in an extremely weak state. Therefore, he was force-fed in accordance with Austrian hospital law. He refused all medical treatment and was given intramuscular sedation against his will. At this time he was attached to a security bed, but he managed to cut through the net and straps. He continued on hunger strike, which caused further deterioration of his physical and mental condition and he was again transferred to a medical intensive care unit.

He was returned to the psychiatric hospital after two weeks, handcuffed and with a belt placed about his ankles because of the continued risk of aggression. Previous physical resistance to forced administrations of antipsychotics had resulted in injuries to him, including loss of teeth, broken ribs and bruises. He remained in these restraints for 15 days but continued his hunger strike and was force-fed. Gradually his physical and mental condition improved and he stopped the hunger strike after a doctor explained to him how the strike was endangering his life.

Mr Herczegfalvy subsequently took the Austrian government to the European Court of Human Rights, alleging that violent and excessively prolonged measures were used to treat him, in violation of article 3 of the ECHR. He also argued that these measures contributed to the worsening of his condition. The judge ruled that the established principles of medicine are admittedly decisive in such cases, *but concluded,* as a general rule, a measure which is a therapeutic necessity cannot be regarded as inhuman or degrading *and the Court must satisfy itself that such medical necessity has been convincingly shown to exist. The Court accepted that, according to psychiatric principles generally accepted at the time, medical necessity justified the treatment at issue and therefore there had been no violation of article 3.*

The above case study clearly demonstrates that inhuman or degrading treatment can be interpreted in a number of ways that are dependent on the unique circumstances of each case. In many ways, the treatment of Mr Herczegfalvy could be considered as harsh and degrading. However, the sole aim and focus was therapeutic. Therefore, the judge ruled that article 3 was not applicable in his case.

Article 8

This article states:

1. *Everyone has the right to respect for his private and family life, his home and his correspondence.*
2. *There shall be no interference by a public authority with the exercise of this right except such as is in accordance with the law and is necessary in a democratic society in the interests of national security, public safety or the economic well-being of the country, for the prevention of disorder or crime, for the protection of health or morals, or for the protection of the rights and freedoms of others.*

The key area of article 8 is to protect the individual's right to privacy, and prevent a public authority from intruding unnecessarily into a person's private life. For example, article 8 may be breached, in some cases, where people are subjected to undue surveillance, or the interception of their telephone calls, or the publication of newspaper accounts of their private life. Article 8 also protects rights to family life, which means that decisions regarding custody or adoption must take into account the rights to family life of all those involved. It also protects the individual's right to physical integrity, and the right to respect for their home.

Article 8 has been one of the most dynamically applied provisions of the ECHR. It has an extremely wide application, for example the use of medical records in court, or the right to practise one's sexuality.

Activity 2.3   *Evidence-based practice and research*

A patient detained under section 3 of the Mental Health Act 1983 complained that his human rights under articles 8 and 3 of the ECHR had been breached because he was made to take antipsychotic medication that had unpleasant side effects.

- Can you explain why both articles 8 and 3 may be relevant in this case?
- What do you think was the outcome of the case?

Outline answers are provided at the end of the chapter.

Article 8 has been used to assess such common, everyday issues as the provision of personal care by same-gender staff, assistance to move to suitably adapted accommodation and the appropriate use of bedpans, and also complex, end-of-life decisions. Because of the nature of article 8 it will continue to be tested in many and varied clinical situations and also in the area of research.

Mental Capacity Act 2005

This Act covers all personal decisions on the welfare of people who temporarily or permanently lack mental capacity to decide for themselves. It defines someone as lacking in capacity if:

at the time, he [sic] is unable to make a decision for himself because of an impairment of, or a disturbance in the functioning of, the mind or brain.

The first section of the Act outlines five principles that are designed to protect people who lack capacity to make their own decisions, and also to maximise people's ability to make their own decisions as far as they are capable of doing so.

1. An individual must be assumed to have capacity unless it is determined otherwise.
2. An individual is not to be regarded as unable to make a decision unless all practicable steps to help the individual to do so have been taken without success.
3. An individual is not to be regarded as unable to make a decision merely because he or she makes an unwise decision.
4. An act done or a decision made under the Act, for or on behalf of a person who lacks capacity, must be done in his or her best interests.
5. Before the act is done, or the decision is made, consideration must be given as to whether the purpose for which the decision or act is needed can be as effectively achieved in a way that is less restrictive of the person's rights and freedom of action.

The Act enshrines in law best practice and common law principles concerning people who lack mental capacity to decide for themselves and those who take decisions on their behalf. It also deals with the assessment of a person's capacity and those who may act on the patient's behalf. This is done by setting out a clear test to assess whether someone lacks capacity to take a particular decision at a particular time. No one can be labelled 'incapable' simply as a result of a particular medical condition or diagnosis.

In section 2 of the Act, it is clear that a lack of capacity cannot be established merely by reference to a person's age, appearance, or any condition or aspect of a person's behaviour that might lead others to make unjustified assumptions about capacity. A person can put their wishes and feelings into a written statement that can be used as guide at times when that person might lack capacity. Also, people involved in caring for the person lacking capacity have a right to be consulted concerning a person's best interests. Before you read further, please try Activity 2.4.

Activity 2.4   *Critical thinking*

May is a 25-year-old Chemistry graduate who has had numerous admissions to hospital usually on a section order of the Mental Health Act. She suffers from schizophrenia and, on last discharge from hospital, the consultant psychiatrist prescribed a depot injection instead of the usual tablets. The doctor wanted May to break the cycle of hospital admissions by ensuring compliance with medication. May was unhappy about taking a depot injection and argued that she suffers worse side effects on a depot than she does while taking oral medication. The consultant psychiatrist refused May's request, arguing that she has made similar promises in the past without honouring them; in his view she lacked capacity.

*   Does May lack capacity?
*   What other factors might be leading May to refuse medication?

Outline answers are provided at the end of the chapter.

Section 5 of the Act offers legal protection from liability where a person is performing an act in connection with the care or treatment of someone who lacks capacity. This could cover actions that might otherwise attract criminal prosecution or civil liability if someone has to interfere with the person's body or property in the course of providing care or treatment.

Section 6 of the Act defines restraint as:

> *the use or threat of force where a person who lacks capacity resists, and any restriction of liberty or movement whether or not the person resists.*

Restraint is only permitted if the person using it reasonably believes it is necessary to prevent harm to the person who lacks capacity, and if the restraint used is a proportionate response to the likelihood and seriousness of the harm.

Scenario

Mr Jones is 73 years old, lives in the community on his own and has no known living relatives; he is showing early signs of Alzheimer's disease. A care worker visits daily to ensure his needs are attended to. Recently, the care worker has noticed a deterioration in Mr Jones's level of coping with activities of daily living, and a care conference has been arranged to make an application to the court to appoint a person to make decisions on his behalf and look after his welfare.

The Mental Capacity Act 2005 allows a person to appoint an attorney to act on their behalf if they should lose capacity in the future. In addition, it provides for a system of court-appointed deputies to take decisions on welfare, healthcare and financial matters as authorised by the Court of Protection, but the appointee will not be able to refuse consent to life-sustaining treatment on behalf of the patient.

In addition to the above, the Act provides for an Independent Mental Capacity Advocate (IMCA), who is appointed to support a person who lacks capacity but has no one, such as family or friends, to speak for them. The IMCA will only be involved where decisions are being made about serious medical treatment or a change in the person's accommodation where it is provided by the NHS or a local authority. The IMCA makes representations about the person's wishes, feelings, beliefs and values, at the same time as bringing to the attention of the decision maker all factors that are relevant to the decision. The IMCA can challenge the decision maker on behalf of the person lacking capacity, if necessary.

Mental Health Act 1983 (amended)

This Act, which was amended in 2007, is mainly concerned with the circumstances in which a person with a mental health problem can be detained for treatment for that condition without their consent. There is procedure that must be followed in order to safeguard patients from inappropriate detention or treatment without consent. In summary, the legislation ensures that people with serious mental disorders that threaten their health and safety, or the safety of the public, can be treated, if necessary, without their consent. This is to prevent them from harming themselves or others. In medicines management, we are mainly concerned with sections 2, 3, and 37.

Section 2

> ## Case study
>
> *Yosuf is a 36-year-old man with no history of mental health problems. After the death of his mother nine months ago, he became withdrawn. His appetite and sleep pattern deteriorated. He denied experiencing any mental health problems but admits to hearing the voice of his mother at night. He was recently rushed to hospital after being found unconscious after taking a mixture of alcohol and sleeping tablets. After he regained consciousness in hospital, he asked to be discharged but was referred to the duty psychiatrist. The duty psychiatrist thought Yosuf was suffering from a mental disorder and recommended that he be admitted to a psychiatric unit for assessment under section 2 of the Mental Health Act.*

Section 2 of the Mental Health Act allows compulsory admission for assessment, or for assessment followed by treatment. An application under section 2 can be made by a relative or an Approved Mental Health Professional (AMHP) and must be supported by two medical recommendations. One of the medical recommendations must be from an approved doctor under section 12 of the Act. In practice, the doctor is normally a psychiatrist or a senior registrar with special experience in the diagnosis and treatment of mental disorder.

Both medical recommendations must agree that the detention is in the best interests of the patient, and is for the patient's own safety or that of others. Also, the medical reports should state that the patient is suffering from a mental disorder of a nature or degree that warrants detention for assessment, or assessment followed by treatment. The detention can last up to 28 days and the patient can appeal to the Mental Health Review Tribunal within 14 days of admission. If a patient does not appeal within that period, the patient is automatically referred to a tribunal.

Section 3

> ## Scenario
>
> *Jane has a history of depression, suicidal attempts and abusing alcohol. She has had numerous previous admissions to hospital, usually after taking a drug overdose. She was admitted informally to a ward but she wanted to discharge herself within hours of admission. Because Jane presented a high risk to herself, her consultant psychiatrist recommended that Jane be detained in hospital under section 3 of the Mental Health Act.*

Section 3 is similar to section 2, differing only in that the detention is specifically for treatment and the duration may be up to six months initially and can be extended for another six months, then yearly afterwards. The grounds for detaining a patient under this section are:

- the patient suffers or is suffering from a mental disorder in accordance with the definition of mental disorder in the 2007 amended Mental Health Act;
- it is necessary for the health or safety of the patient or for the protection of other persons, and such treatment cannot be provided unless they are detained under this section.

In addition to the responsible clinician, the written agreement of a second professional is needed to renew section 3. The second professional must:

- come from a different professional discipline than the responsible clinician;
- be involved with the care of the patient;
- be able to reach independent decisions;
- have sufficient expertise and experience to make a judgement about whether the criteria for detention continue to be met.

There may be instances where the responsible clinician disagrees with the view of the second professional and, in such cases, the section 3 detention should not be renewed. In very exceptional circumstances, where there is a difference of opinion, this should be brought to the attention of the hospital managers who are required to consider and approve the renewal of the detention.

The patient has the right to appeal to the Mental Health Review Tribunal within the first six months and then once a year afterwards. As in section 2, the patient will automatically be referred to the Tribunal where a patient themselves has not done so.

Section 37

Section 37 of the Mental Health Act 1983 (amended in 2007) is similar in its application to section 3, but refers specifically to offenders seen before the courts. Appeal against this section can only occur in the second six months of treatment. The discharge of people committed to hospital under this section can be restricted under section 41 of the Act. If a restriction under section 41 is applied, the patient cannot be discharged, granted leave or transferred to another institution without Home Office consent.

Ethical considerations of compulsory treatment

Case study

Owen Perry was convicted of killing five family members in Louisiana, USA. He was sentenced to death but was also found to be suffering from schizophrenia. He believed that Olivia Newton-John was a goddess living under Lake Arthur. On one occasion he shaved his eyebrows, believing that this would allow more oxygen to his brain. The Louisiana District Court ordered Owen Perry to have a depot injection (Haldol) so that his mental condition improved enough to enable him to understand that he would be executed. This decision was later overturned by the Louisiana Supreme Court, leaving Owen Perry untreated and severely psychotic while waiting execution.

Apart from legal considerations, the use of compulsory treatment on people suffering from mental illness has ethical ramifications. For you to understand the origins of compulsory treatment and the moral and ethical issues surrounding it, we need briefly to review earlier work by some anti-psychiatrists, most notably Thomas Szasz. In *Coercion as Cure* (2007), Szasz covers an extensive history of the use of coercion throughout psychiatry, including the early use of various mechanical restraints such as the 'tranquilizing chair', moral treatment, the 'resting cure', insulin shock therapy, electro-convulsive therapy (ECT), lobotomy and, of course, medication. He argues that each one of these breakthrough 'discoveries' in psychiatric medicine is simply a reworking of old ideas, and that all share the common thread of coercion, thus depriving people of their liberty. He further argues that the 'liberation' of patients from mental hospitals by virtue of medicines such as chlorpromazine in the 1950s amounted to no more than drugged coercion, with patients still under compulsory treatment orders in the community. He rejects the use of medicines and coercion in psychiatry altogether, and calls for an abolition of psychiatric coercion as a 'crime against humanity'.

Szasz also makes the point that, in assessing any therapeutic intervention outcome, what should be considered is not its effectiveness but whether it was brought about consensually or coercively. To an extent, Szasz's views inform the absolutist civil liberties approach, whose conviction is that psychiatric hospitalisation of a person against his or her will is a dangerous assault on individual freedom.

Another currently and perhaps more influential civil liberties position is to accept compulsory treatment under certain circumstances but only when exercising extreme caution. Medical necessity is regarded as insufficient reason to justify the use of coercive powers. Only in circumstances where a person is at physical risk of harming him- or herself or others can treatment coercion be applied.

A third view is informed by medicine, which regrets the necessity for involuntary hospitalisation but regards it as an essential last resort, enabling the care and treatment of a small proportion of patients whose severe mental illnesses substantially interfere with their capacity to accept such treatment voluntarily.

As you can imagine, these opposing views evoke lively and polarising debates and this is best exemplified by the case of Owen Perry above. The fact that the district judge and the Supreme Court took differing views that are equally controversial is a case in point. As a nurse you may be caught up in the moral dilemma of patients' needs versus patients' rights, but what is important here is for you to be aware that we are dealing primarily with questions of values not facts. Members of the multidisciplinary team as well as yourself might have different perceptions regarding a particular situation, thus making it very difficult to arrive at a common ground with other members of the team. Clearly, you need to be aware of the ethical dilemmas that may confront you from time to time during the treatment of your patients. You should be assisted by legislation in making decisions and the Medicines Act 1968, discussed shortly, is an important element in medicines management.

Ethical conflicts

There is little doubt that the principle of justice comes into conflict with other ethical considerations in mental health practice. In particular, the principle of autonomy, which focuses on the needs and rights of the individual, gives rise to ethical dilemmas more in mental health than in other fields of nursing. This may be because of the highly patient-oriented approach that is more common in the mental health field (Berghmans et al., 2004). The patient-oriented approach stresses the importance of taking the values and preferences of the individual into account in treatment decisions. For example, Pound et al. (2005) conducted the qualitative equivalent of a meta-analysis of issues surrounding the way in which patients don't take their medication as prescribed. They identified that the concept of 'resistance' to taking medication was linked to the patient's sense of self. Continued taking of psychotropic medication may undermine the feeling of self and therefore may result in less than optimal adherence, despite the obvious benefit the patient derives from taking such medicines. Clearly, this situation generates a conflict in the nurse between, on the one hand, the need to respect patient autonomy and the patient's right to make decisions and, on the other hand, the nurse's duty to promote good mental health through adherence to treatment. In addition to ethical considerations in mental health, you need to be aware of the legislation that specifically governs the use of medicines.

Medicines Act 1968

This important Act, with which you must comply, deals with the prescribing, supply, storage and administration of medicines and defines three categories of medicines:

1. prescription-only medicines (POMs), which are available only from a pharmacist if prescribed by an appropriate practitioner;
2. pharmacy (P) medicines, which are available only from a pharmacist but may be obtained without a prescription;
3. general sales list (GSL) medicines, which may be bought from any shop without a prescription.

Under the Act, possession of prescription medicines such as antibiotics, with or without a prescription, is not a specified offence. Possession of a POM without a prescription is only an offence if the drug is also controlled under the Misuse of Drugs Act 1971.

Misuse of Drugs Act 1971

The main purpose of this Act is to prevent the non-medical use of certain medicines or drugs. It achieves this by imposing a complete ban on the possession, supply, manufacture, import and export of controlled drugs (CDs), except as allowed by regulations or licence from the Secretary of State. In addition to banning the possession of illegal drugs, the Act prohibits their import, export, production and supply. It also makes it illegal to incite another person to do any of the above. It is also an offence to knowingly allow premises to be used for drug misuse. Under the Act, cannabis plant cultivation, possession of opium pipes and the possession of hypodermic syringes for illegal drug injection are all banned. Initially, the Act divides drugs into three classes – A, B and C.

- **Class A** includes heroin, cocaine, crack, LSD, ecstasy, 'magic mushrooms', morphine and amphetamines for injection. The penalty for possession of these drugs can be an unlimited fine and/or up to seven years in prison. The penalty for dealing can be an unlimited fine and/or up to life in prison.
- **Class B** includes cannabis, dihydrocodeine, methylphenidate (Ritalin), pholcodine and amphetamines. The penalty for possession of these drugs can be an unlimited fine and/or up to five years in prison and, for dealing in these drugs, an unlimited fine and/or up to 14 years in prison.
- **Class C** includes anabolic steroids, benzodiazepines, gammahydroxybutyrate (GHB) and ketamine. The penalty for possession can be an unlimited fine and/or up to two years in prison. For dealing class C drugs, the penalty can be an unlimited fine and/or up to 14 years in prison.

Because most CDs have medical uses or are of scientific interest, the Act allows the government to authorise possession, supply, production and import or export of drugs to meet medical or scientific needs. These exemptions are expressed in the form of 'regulations' made under the Act. CDs are classified as follows.

- **Schedule 1**. These drugs are the most stringently controlled. They are not authorised for medical use and can only be supplied, possessed or administered in exceptional circumstances under a special Home Office licence, usually only for research purposes. Examples include cannabis, coca leaf, ecstasy, LSD, raw opium and psilocin.
- **Schedules 2 and 3** drugs are available for medical use and can be prescribed by doctors. It is illegal to be in possession of these drugs without a doctor's prescription. Schedule 2 drugs include amphetamines, cocaine, dihydrocodeine, Diconal, heroin, methadone, morphine, opium in medicinal form, pethidine and Ritalin and are subject to strict record keeping and storage in pharmacies. Schedule 3 drugs include barbiturates, Rohypnol and temazepam tranquillisers and are subject to restrictions on prescription writing.
- **Schedule 4** has recently been divided into two parts. Part 1 comprises most minor tranquillisers (other than Rohypnol and temazepam) and eight other substances. It is now illegal to be in possession of these minor tranquillisers without a prescription. Part 2 comprises anabolic steroids, which can be legally possessed in medicinal form without a prescription but which it is illegal to supply to other people.
- **Schedule 5** drugs are considered to pose minimal risk of abuse. Some of these are dilute, small-dose, non-injectable preparations that are allowed to be sold over the counter at a pharmacy without a prescription, and all may be possessed by anyone. But once bought they cannot be legally supplied to another person. Among these are some well-known cough medicines, anti-diarrhoea agents and mild painkillers.

An understanding of the Misuse of Drugs Act is important in the administration of medicines as well as in prescribing.

Medicinal Products: Prescription by Nurses etc. Act 1992

Non-medical prescribing relates to prescribing by professional groups, other than doctors or dentists, who have been granted prescribing rights. These professionals include nurses, pharmacists, optometrists, midwives and health visitors. In 1992 the Medicinal Products: Prescription by Nurses etc. Act was passed, leading to amendments of the Medicines Act 1968 and the NHS Act 1977. The Act came about as a result of the changes in healthcare and the realisation that there could be significant benefits to nurses having prescribing rights. These rights were extended initially only to community nurses. There are two types of prescribers: independent prescribers, who would be responsible for the assessment of patients with undiagnosed conditions and for making decisions about the clinical management of these patients; and supplementary prescribers, who would be responsible for the continuing care of patients who have been clinically assessed by an independent prescriber.

Supplementary prescribing

Supplementary prescribing involves a voluntary partnership between an independent prescriber, who must be a doctor or dentist, and a supplementary prescriber to implement an agreed patient-specific clinical management plan (CMP) with the patient's agreement. Supplementary prescribing has two tiers: doctors or dentists ('independent prescribers') are responsible for the diagnosis of the patient, and for determining the type of medicines that may be prescribed by the supplementary prescriber under a CMP for the patient; and other health professionals ('supplementary prescribers') who are responsible for the continuing care of the patient in accordance with a CMP. They have authority to prescribe specific medicines for particular medical conditions in accordance with the plan. According to the Department of Health (**www.dh.gov.uk**), the supplementary prescribing programme is designed *to ease the burden on doctors and improve access to medicines*.

Supplementary prescribing starts with an agreed CMP, which is mandatory and must be clearly documented in the patient's notes. A CMP is defined as a written plan relating to the treatment of a patient as agreed by: (a) the relevant patient, (b) the doctor who is the independent prescriber and (c) any supplementary prescriber who is to prescribe, give directions for administration or administer under the plan. The plan may be amended from time to time.

Nurse supplementary prescribers can prescribe any medicines that are listed in an agreed CMP. These medicines include:

- GSL medicines, P medicines or POMs;
- antibiotics and antifungal, antiprotozoa and antiviral medicines;
- medicines that are new to the market or require intensive surveillance; these drugs are generally referred to as 'black triangle' medicines;
- products used outside their UK licensed indications (off-label use). Such use must have the joint agreement of both prescribers and the status of the drug should be recorded in the CMP.

There are no legal restrictions on the clinical conditions that may be dealt with by a supplementary prescriber. The DH advises that supplementary prescribing is primarily intended for use in managing specific long-term medical conditions or health needs affecting the patient. However, acute episodes occurring within long-term conditions may be included in these arrangements, provided they are included in the CMP.

Independent prescribing

Nurses who have undertaken further training are able to independently prescribe from a larger range of medicines. Any first-level nurses or a registered midwife may take further training to be an independent prescriber. The *Nurse Prescribers' Extended Formulary* (NPEF) was introduced in 2002 and has been expanded several times, the last being in 2005 to cover an extended range of medicines and conditions outside the original therapeutic areas, mainly for emergency care and first-contact care.

Patient group directions

Patient group directions (PGDs) are documents that make it legal for medicines to be given to groups of patients without individual prescriptions having to be written for each patient. They can also be used to empower staff other than doctors (for example, nurses and paramedics) to give the medicine in question legally. For example, a nurse could supply an asthma inhaler or administer flu vaccine to a patient without the need for a prescription or an instruction from a prescriber.

However, for a PGD to be valid, certain criteria must be met in terms of the patient group, what the PGD can be used for and how the PGD itself is drawn up. Organisations also have a responsibility to ensure that only fully competent, trained healthcare professionals use PGDs. A PGD must be signed by a senior doctor and a pharmacist, both of whom should have been involved in developing the direction. Additionally, the PGD must be authorised by the relevant appropriate body as set out in the legislation.

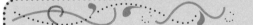

Chapter summary

As a nurse, you play an extremely critical role in people's lives, particularly at times when they are most vulnerable. The decisions you make as a nurse can have a long-term impact on people's physical and mental health. For this reason, it is only proper that you should be accountable for your actions and omissions. There is a plethora of legislation that regulates the way you practise as a nurse, such as that based on the European Convention on Human Rights, which states that every human being is entitled to life; that no one should be subjected to degrading and inhuman treatment; and that everyone has a right to privacy. The Mental Capacity Act 2005 gives recognition to the view that everyone should be regarded as mentally capable of deciding for themselves unless proved otherwise. Further, if someone lacks capacity, a procedure for appointing someone to act on behalf of the individual ought to be followed. This Act is closely linked to sections of the Mental Health Act 1983 (amended), which states that treatment can be given to people against their will should particular criteria be satisfied.

continued . . .

> With regard to legislation that deals with the supply and administering of medicines, the Medicines Act 1968 classifies medicines depending on whether a person requires a prescription or not to obtain them. It is not an offence under this Act to be in possession of prescription-only medicines. However, it is an offence to be in possession of controlled drugs without a prescription under the Misuse of Drugs Act 1971.

Activities: brief outline answers

Activity 2.1 Breach of the Human Rights Act 1998 (page 43)

The answer is 'Yes'. To breach article 2, death does not necessarily need to occur. Although hospital policy and good practice states that vital signs should be recorded regularly if someone is administered intramuscular or intravenous antipsychotic medication, this was not done, therefore putting the patient at material risk. This alone is sufficient to breach article 2 of the Human Rights Act.

Activity 2.3 Breach of the Mental Health Act 1983 (page 46)

Article 8 has been breached because the patient had no choice of medication. Article 3 has been breached because of the imposition of antipsychotic drugs resulting in unpleasant side effects.

The outcome was that the case was dismissed because, even if the medical treatment in question and the applicant's lack of choice of therapist had breached Article 8(1), this could be justified under Article 8(2) because of the need to maintain public order and to protect the applicant's own health. As for the patient suffering unpleasant side effects, the patient is not protected under article 3 because the purpose of giving antipsychotics to the patient was not to inflict side effects but to treat a psychiatric condition that the patient suffered from.

Activity 2.4 Lack of capacity (page 47)

It is unlikely that May lacks capacity; she appears to understand that she needs medication, but it does appear that she is not involved in the decision-making process, and it is therefore not surprising that May finds ways of avoiding medication. The issue of side effects and how to manage them may be impacting on her willingness to take medication.

Further reading

Griffith, R and Tengnah, C (2010) *Law and Professional Issues in Nursing* (2nd edition). Exeter: Learning Matters.

This is a very useful book that covers most aspects of nursing practice law.

Department of Health (1983) Mental Health Act 1983. Available online at www.legislation.gov.uk.

This is the government publication of the entire Act.

Useful websites

www.the-shipman-inquiry.org.uk

Harold Shipman was a general practitioner who murdered his patients and this inquiry into his conduct sets out recommendations.

Chapter 3
The therapeutic alliance and the promotion of adherence to medication

Chapter aims

By the end of this chapter, you should be able to:

* understand the concept of adherence and associated problems;
* outline factors that mediate adherence to medication;

- explain illness perceptions and health-seeking behaviours;
- understand the therapeutic alliance and its development;
- describe strategies for improving adherence and readiness to change;
- understand the concept of shared decision-making.

Introduction

The treatment of psychological problems goes as far back as the fifth century BC when mental disorders, particularly psychotic disorders, were considered supernatural in origin. This view was prevalent during both Greek and Roman times, but early writings in the fourth century BC suggest that, even then, the role of biology in mental disorders was recognised, particularly by Hippocrates. However, religious leaders and others who were powerful at the time continued to use forms of exorcism to treat mental disorders and these methods were often barbaric. It was not until the medieval age that care for the mentally ill significantly changed.

In medieval Europe, psychiatric hospitals were built from the thirteenth century to treat mental disorders, but were used only as custodial institutions and did not provide any type of treatment. In complete contrast to the prevailing Christian approach, which relied on demonological explanations for mental illness, the medieval Muslim approach was based mostly on clinical observations. Records also show that Muslims were among the first to provide psychotherapy and moral treatment for those who were mentally ill. Other forms of treatment included baths, drug medication, music therapy and occupational therapy. In the Western world, it was not until the early 1950s that there was a dramatic change in the treatment and care of people with mental disorders and particularly those with psychosis. This was mainly due to the discovery of anti-psychotic medication.

The introduction of psychiatric medications altered the relationship between mental health professionals and their patients. This shift was interpreted as a lack of concern for patients and this, in part, gave birth to an 'anti-psychiatry movement' in the late twentieth century. This was also due to the much-publicised view that mental illness was a myth and psychiatry was a form of social control; the movement demanded that institutionalised psychiatric care be abolished. Although the popularity of the anti-psychiatry movement has declined, it had the positive outcome of helping mental health professionals become more sensitive to the needs of those with mental health problems.

Now we turn to the role of the nurse in the care of people with mental illness.

The history of the mental health nurse

While the formal recognition of psychiatry occurred early in the nineteenth century with the development of the modern cognitive sciences, psychiatric nursing as a profession was not recognised until the latter part of the century. As with psychiatry in general, mental health nursing suffered from many misinformed theories of cognition and mental illness, leading to practices that would now be deemed counterproductive or even harmful. Subsequent advances in cognition and psychology produced a more balanced approach that combined medical procedures, medicines and cognitive therapy in order to improve the mental health of the individual. Mental health nursing, in particular, had difficulties with the shifting environment of the mental health profession, often being caught between competing viewpoints, and this has been reflected in the debate regarding the 'medical model' and the 'psychological model'.

Where available, care has tended to become more intimate and holistic, taking various approaches and applying them where applicable to the complete person. This has brought the concept of medication adherence and the **therapeutic alliance** into being.

This chapter will initially explore the concept of medication adherence before dealing with issues relating to forming an effective therapeutic alliance. The importance of a therapeutic alliance in promoting treatment and recovery will be covered before dealing with strategies for improving patient adherence to medication. The final sections will cover what the patient needs to know and common errors that occur during the formation of a therapeutic alliance.

Medication adherence

Early conceptions of medication adherence originate from the authoritarian, traditional medical model, which equated adherence with compliance. A more recent conceptualisation involves medication adherence as a **collaborative process** where the patient is included and is an active participant in their own treatment (Berk et al., 2004). This concept of adherence places the therapeutic alliance at the heart of the process and uses the relationship as the vehicle for exchanging information and opening up discussion aimed at reaching a 'concordance' about treatment. The concept of **concordance** will be explained in later sections.

From a practical aspect, adherence involves a number of behaviours that include accessing treatment, obtaining medications, understanding and following instructions about taking medications and remembering to take medications. When the person intentionally decides not to adhere to treatment, non-adherence is said to be voluntary, and it is involuntary where the lack of adherence is unintentional. An example of involuntary non-adherence is when a patient forgets to take their medication.

You may observe that some patients may modify, rather than completely accept or abandon treatment. This behaviour is called *partial adherence*. For example, a patient may only take part of their full dose, or may stop and restart treatment sporadically for varying intervals.

Another form of non-adherence is *over-adherence* through possible abuse of prescription medication. An example of this is where a patient is only required to take one tablet, but instead takes three. This is particularly common in people who are prescribed anti-anxiety or pain-relief medicines. A further form of adherence behaviour is *selective adherence*. This is when a patient may choose to be fully adherent to one type of medicine and non-adherent to another. A good example of selective adherence is the person who suffers from depression and diabetes, who is fully adherent to medicines for diabetes but is not adherent to antidepressants. You can see from these examples that adherence is a dynamic and changing process that varies in a number of ways. This is why the nurse needs to discuss adherence with the patient repeatedly throughout the treatment process. However, to determine the extent of adherence is a difficult task that will be discussed in a later section. In spite of the challenge posed by the measurement of adherence, its importance in the treatment and recovery of people with mental health problems is clear, and it is this that we will discuss next.

The importance of medication adherence

There is sufficient research evidence to suggest that medication plays a crucial role in determining the outcome and recovery of people suffering from all types of illnesses and this is also true for those suffering from mental health problems. As such, treatment with **psychotropic medication** plays a pivotal role despite advances in other forms of treatment. There is also evidence to suggest that non-adherence to medication is a widespread problem in all types of illness, including mental illness. Relapse of illness due to non-adherence has many personal, social and economic consequences, particularly for those suffering from mental health problems.

Relapse causes patients to suffer distressing symptoms that can lead to hospitalisation. In turn, hospitalisation usually results in disruption to the patient's life and this can lead to a family losing income, particularly if the patient is the wage earner (Bebbington, 1995). In this regard, Becker and Maiman (1975) have suggested that unsuccessful management of medication adherence is related to poor clinical response and may be the most common cause of illness relapse, which increases treatment costs. For example, Knapp et al. (2004) estimated the annual total cost of patient hospitalisation to be upwards of £5,000 per patient per year in people suffering from schizophrenia alone. In the treatment of people with psychosis, evidence suggests that the intermittent pattern of medication-taking associated with non-adherence increases the incidence of **tardive dyskinesia** (see Chapter 7). Further, prolonged, untreated psychosis may diminish the effectiveness of medication treatment, and other researchers have noted that non-adherence to medication is associated with longer hospitalisations and increased suicidal behaviour (Qurashi et al., 2006).

From a social perspective, relapse caused by non-adherence in people with psychosis may be more dangerous than relapse that occurs while a patient is taking medication, being more severe and disruptive (Torrey, 1994). Despite the importance of medication adherence in the treatment of people with mental health problems, it has not so far been possible to introduce an accurate way of measuring it. We now look at possible solutions to this problem.

The measurement of adherence

We now know that adherence to medication is not 'all or nothing' and may be partial, irregular or selective. This poses a challenge to nurses who need to estimate adherence accurately, but currently there is no universally agreed method of doing this. Current methods of assessing adherence include:

- patient self-reports;
- reports by family members or significant others;

- biological tests;
- pill counts;
- pharmacy refill records;
- electronic methods.

All these methods have limitations; for example, it has been suggested that self-reporting by patients is potentially unreliable, as patients may overestimate or over-report their treatment adherence. In the case of using blood plasma levels of the medicine as a measure of adherence, adherence to long **half-life** medicines, such as antipsychotics, may be overestimated. Also, the assessment of some medicines with great inter-individual variations of serum levels, such as antidepressants, would be confusing. Although electronic medication packs may provide more reliable information about adherence, associated costs tend to be prohibitive for use in clinical practice. Information from pill count assessments may be unreliable as patients may not necessarily be ingesting the pills after removing them from packaging.

Clearly, the estimation of adherence is difficult and the concept of adherence is shaped by an individual's health belief system. But before you proceed, you may wish to work on Activity 3.1.

Activity 3.1   *Reflection*

In a group or on your own, discuss and list reasons why a patient may decide to be partially adherent to medication.

An outline answer is provided at the end of the chapter.

Health beliefs and health-seeking behaviour

Health-seeking behaviour has been defined as any action undertaken by individuals who perceive they have a health problem for the purpose of finding an appropriate remedy. The behaviour starts with a decision-making process that is dependent on an individual's family, community values and expectations. It is also controlled by the characteristics and behaviour of the health provider. These factors interact to produce a final choice of a health-seeking option that may typically involve recognition of symptoms and the perceived nature of the illness, followed by appropriate care and monitoring.

Several theories that seek to explain health-seeking behaviour have been proposed. We will now look at the most common, which are the biomedical and health belief models.

The biomedical model

Early biomedical theories were couched in terms of the institutionally defined roles of 'authority' and 'supplicant' (the patient). In other words, in this approach the doctor prescribes, and the patient complies with the medication regimen. This autocratic outlook viewed non-adherence as a failing of the patient through lack of knowledge, motivation and will. You will occasionally witness vestiges of this approach, particularly when people use expressions such as 'the patient failed the treatment', but these biases are not usually supported by research evidence because, as you will see later, no specific patient characteristic consistently relates to non-adherence behaviour.

Despite obvious flaws in the biomedical model, it has several aspects that we may find useful. First, it makes a critical contribution to the concept of adherence by specifying a number of factors that impact on medication adherence. Among these is the prescribed treatment regimen as the criterion against which adherence behaviour is to be evaluated. The biomedical model also focuses on medication side effects as undesirable outcomes that affect medication adherence and efficacy. The biomedical model has endured in the face of other models that potentially have more explanatory value. One such model is the health belief model.

The health belief model

The health belief model (HBM) was first developed in the 1950s by social psychologists Hochbaum, Rosenstock and Kegels, working in the US Public Health Services. It was developed in response to the failure of a free tuberculosis health screening programme and, since then, the HBM has been adapted to explore a variety of long- and short-term health behaviours, including sexual risk behaviours and the transmission of HIV/AIDS. It attempts to explain and predict health behaviours of people by focusing on the attitudes and beliefs of individuals. It considers five main areas that are likely to influence health-seeking behaviour. Put simply, from the patient's viewpoint, these are as follows.

- Perceived susceptibility: Am I going to get the disease?
- Perceived seriousness: How bad would it be?
- Perceived benefits and barriers: How easy would it be to get something done about it? What is it going to cost me?
- Self-efficacy: Am I able to make any changes?
- Cues to action: OK, now I am going to do something about it!

Perceived susceptibility

For a given condition, a patient will have a perception of how susceptible they are to developing the illness. This perception might be based on experience: they might have a parent or sibling with the disease and therefore convince themselves that they too will get it. Conversely, they may feel that they are somehow invulnerable to certain diseases. For example, we all come across a smoker who refuses to give up because they know a lifelong smoker who has never had any health problems. Another important factor that shapes perceived susceptibility is awareness of illness and this is particularly relevant in people with psychosis. When someone believes they are not suffering from a particular illness, they are unlikely to feel susceptible to it despite the presence of symptoms, and may offer an alternative explanation for these symptoms.

Perceived seriousness

Patients differ in how serious they consider different conditions to be, and this interacts with their perception of susceptibility. For instance, a patient may be at low risk of developing bowel cancer, but since they perceive it as a very serious condition, may feel motivated to see the doctor about persistent loose stools. Another patient may consider a headache a triviality, and feel that seeing the doctor would be a waste of the doctor's time, and therefore possibly fail to have a serious condition diagnosed.

Perception of seriousness can affect not only whether or not a patient presents to a healthcare service, but also *where* they present. If a patient feels that coughing up green phlegm is serious they may consult their doctor, but if they consider it trivial, they may take the problem to a pharmacist. This last point is important because it also interacts with cultural factors. Try Activity 3.2 before proceeding further.

Activity 3.2   *Critical thinking*

Julio is a 33-year-old man who has a long history of reluctance to seek help from psychiatric services even though he suffers from an unspecified psychotic illness. Although Julio acknowledges that he becomes unwell, he believes that this is due to a jealous relative who cast an evil spell on him when he was a child in South America. He has on several occasions travelled to South America to see a traditional healer who 'exorcised' the evil spirit.

• Is Julio's view of his condition invalid?

An outline answer is provided at the end of the chapter.

Perceived benefits and barriers

Quite often, patients face different options in choosing how to deal with their health concerns. They will often weigh up the potential benefits and drawbacks to each course of action and consider any perceived potential barriers to health-seeking activity. How patients decide which route to take, and the importance they attach to individual benefits, disadvantages and barriers, may differ markedly from person to person.

Self-efficacy

Self-efficacy is a term used to describe how people view their own ability to carry out a particular action. It is defined as *people's beliefs about their capabilities to exercise control over events that affect their lives [and their] beliefs in their capabilities to mobilise the motivation, cognitive resources, and courses of action needed to exercise control over task demands* (Bandura, 1991). Therefore, self-efficacy attributions are concerned *not with the skills one has but with the judgements of what one can do with whatever skills one possesses*. This includes a patient's perception of how likely they are to change particular behaviours. For example, a particular patient may well realise that if he continues smoking he may well get, and die from, heart disease. He has spoken with his GP about this many times and has been offered treatment to stop smoking. He just thinks that he will never be able to stop smoking, so does not think it worth the bother seeking help to stop. A perception of low self-efficacy is the barrier to taking action in this case.

Cues to action

Even when a patient has developed a perception about their health, there usually exists a trigger that turns this into action. From a communication viewpoint, you as the nurse will want to uncover what triggered a patient to seek healthcare. The possible triggers may be quite varied: the media, a relative, an overheard conversation or a reminder letter. Such a prompt may increase a patient's perception of their susceptibility to a disease or of its seriousness; it may remind them of the increased benefits of seeking healthcare. The prompt may increase their motivation to change, or convince them that they may in fact be able to make any required changes themselves. Like all theoretical models, the HBM has some limitations. For this reason, it has been modified over time and the influence of culture, society and the media, as well as demographic factors, are important modifiers that should be considered. Other health-seeking models based on illness perception have been formulated.

The self-regulatory model

The basis of illness perception models in mental health is the self-regulatory model (SRM) (Leventhal et al., 1984). In turn, the SRM is built on at least four components.

- People are active problem solvers and they strive to make sense of their worlds as they search for suitable, effective ways of controlling and adapting to their world.
- People's conceptualisations of health threats are generated by a multi-level processing system, one level being emotional and another intellectual.
- Emotional reactions and the intellectual notions of a disease and its treatment are generated more or less simultaneously.
- Contextual factors including cultural, environmental, social relationships and personality dispositions influence the way individuals understand health threats and how they manage them.

The SRM is currently one of the most widely used models because of its reliability and **validity** in exploring important patient beliefs across a range of physical illnesses, and this has enabled advances to be made in understanding self-management of and recovery from illnesses. The wide applicability of this model suggests that it may be appropriate for both mental and physical illness. Much of the work carried out in mental illness is consistent with this model.

As previously mentioned, the SRM was conceptualised by Leventhal and colleagues in the late 1970s, when they examined how fear messages in relatively acute situations might lead people to take health-promoting actions, such as wearing seat belts or giving up smoking. Leventhal et al. (1984) found that different types of information were needed to influence attitudes and actions to a perceived threat to health and well-being. The SRM proposes that, during illness, two parallel processes are in operation: first, the intellectual or objective interpretation of the threat to health and, second, the emotional or subjective reaction to the threat to health. These parallel processes of intellect and emotion are interactive. For example, adherence to medication in mental health includes intellectual processing of information to understand the complex relationship between medication adherence and the diminishing of symptoms. However, socioculturally related emotional values about illness and medication-taking experiences may be more important than intellectual processes. In such situations, people may choose not to take medication because they feel socially obliged not do so. Before you proceed further, you need to undertake Activity 3.3.

Activity 3.3   *Reflection*

Alone or in a group, think of a situation where a person recognises that he or she is ill but decides not to seek treatment. It may be that you have been in this position yourself.

•   What factors might be influencing the person not to seek treatment?

An outline answer is provided at the end of the chapter.

The key beliefs identified in the SRM refer to a specific illness episode rather than to intellectual beliefs about a possible illness. In applying the SRM to physical illness, five specific components have been identified as key to guiding individual reaction to a threat to health. The original four are:

•   the perceived identity of the illness (including a label and signs/symptoms);
•   the perceived consequences (physical, social and behavioural);
•   the likely causes of the illness;
•   the likely timeline or sense of how long the illness will last.

A fifth belief about the potential for control or cure of the illness has also been added to the model (Lau et al., 1989).

Although originally developed around physical illness, this model could be usefully applied to mental health situations. A good example is that of hypochondriasis. This condition originates when an individual believes they have an illness in response to perceived bodily sensations. The individual's viewpoint is that they have a serious illness, but medical investigations do not confirm this and the medical practitioner's view is that the patient is experiencing anxiety. Repeated reassurance does not work in the long term because it fails to provide the individual with an alternative coherent argument that explains why they experience the bodily sensations. Until this is done, re-experiencing the bodily sensations will trigger the old belief in the illness and the accompanying concern.

There has been considerable support for the model since its inception. For example, how an individual summarises and labels these experiences may have an important impact on their responses and this is linked to perceived quality of life. Mechanic et al. (1994) found that people who attributed their mental illness to a physical, medical or biological problem, as opposed to psychological problems, scored higher on a perceived quality of life measure, and reported less personal stigma and greater self-esteem. Also, the dimension of the likely consequences of having a health problem on their daily lives is related to variations in coping levels, depression and medication adherence.

Patients suffering from schizophrenia, for example, are able to identify strategies they use to cope with their symptoms. Their beliefs about the likely consequences of symptoms appear to influence this relationship. For example, Kinney (1999) showed that patients who perceived their symptoms as more taxing and burdensome were more likely to report difficulties in coping.

Overall, evidence suggests that the SRM is a potentially useful way to understand health-seeking behaviour, although this approach may require modifications before it can usefully be employed in people suffering from psychosis. For example, Kinderman and Bentall (1996) reported that patients experiencing psychosis did not identify their experiences as separate 'illnesses' and did not have 'illness beliefs'. Those patients who are in remission conceptualised their experiences as separate from their normal behaviour and used a conceptual framework that differed significantly from conventional health belief models.

Finally, it is important for you to recognise that the illness models used to increase our understanding of people's responses to mental health problems are theoretical. They are tools to help us in potentially important areas of intervention. These conceptualisations have limitations and cannot replace an individual's perception of illness, which provides a far more complex and useful guide to understanding their illness and what it means for them. If we integrate health-seeking behaviour theories in our understanding of adherence to psychotropic medicines, it is possible to divide factors that pertain to adherence into three broad areas: those that pertain to the patient, those that are illness-related and those that are treatment-related.

Factors influencing adherence

If we integrate the role of health belief and illness perception models, we can see that adherence is a complex behavioural process strongly influenced by the environments in which people live, healthcare providers practise, and healthcare systems deliver care. It is also related to people's knowledge and beliefs about their illness, motivation to manage it, confidence in their ability to engage in illness-management behaviours, and expectations regarding the outcome of treatment and the consequences of poor adherence.

It is important for a nurse to recognise that a person may have multiple risk factors for medication non-adherence. Also, factors that can influence a person's medication-taking behaviour may change over time. You will need to assess a person's adherence throughout their course of treatment. Furthermore, because there is usually no single reason for non-adherence, there can be no 'one size fits all' approach to improving adherence. Before we can discuss strategies for enhancing medication adherence, we need to discuss factors that have been identified to predict adherence.

Illness-related factors

In mental health there is consistent evidence supporting the link between adherence to and severity of illness, called 'condition-related factors' in Figure 3.1. For example, in those suffering from psychotic illness, the severity of symptoms such as paranoia, hostility and delusional beliefs has been linked to poor adherence to medication. One of the earliest studies to identify this link was by Van Putten et al. (1976), who identified the severity of grandiose delusions as particularly predictive of poor adherence. Additionally, it makes sense that people with more severe negative

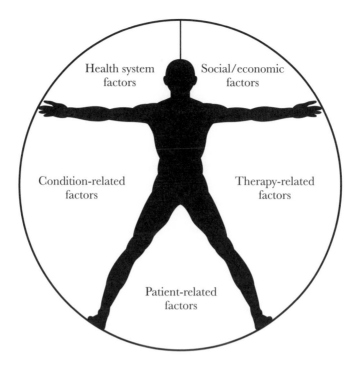

Figure 3.1: The factors associated with adherence to medication (adapted from WHO, 2003, p27)

symptoms, such as impaired motivation, are likely to be non-adherent to medication, and this has been empirically verified (Frangou et al., 2005; Rosa et al., 2005; Yamada et al., 2006;). Yamada et al. (2006) investigated factors implicated in adherence to antipsychotic medication. The investigators found that patients who were more adherent had less severe symptoms than those who were non-adherent. Thus, in general and across a wide range of mental illnesses, the severity of illness is associated with poor medication adherence.

Awareness of illness (insight) and adherence

Activity 3.4 *Critical thinking*

Chris is a 41-year-old man who believes he has telepathic powers and does not like watching television because he can hear his name being discussed on the TV. From time to time, he says he hears the voice of God telling him to leave his flat and sleep on the streets. He does not believe that he suffers from a mental illness and therefore is reluctant to take medication.

• Can you suggest factors that may lead someone to think they have no mental health problems despite evidence to the contrary?

An outline answer is provided at the end of the chapter.

In people with psychosis, an awareness of illness or **insight** has been identified as a predictive factor for adherence behaviour. One of the earliest studies to establish a link between poor insight and medication adherence was in 1988 by Bartkó and colleagues. They found that 55 per cent of the patients in their study who became non-adherent to medication had poor insight. Since this early finding, subsequent work has consistently supported the link between poor insight and poor medication adherence. This relationship has been studied in a wide variety of settings, such as at hospital admission, on discharge, post-discharge and in outpatient clinics.

In summary, poor awareness of illness is recognised as a good indicator that patients will have poor medication adherence, especially those suffering from a psychotic illness.

Adverse side effects and adherence

Many medicines used to treat mental health problems, although effective at controlling symptoms, have adverse side effects, making many patients reluctant to take medication. The problem of non-adherence due to adverse side effects is probably more acute in people suffering from a psychosis. In particular, older or conventional antipsychotic medicines such as chlorpromazine, haloperidol and clopixol are known to cause a wide variety of adverse side effects (see Chapter 7). In people suffering from depression, antidepressant side effects such as sedation, sexual dysfunction and dry mouth can influence whether people take medicines or not. In some situations, patients may not be willing to take medication because of how they function or feel while doing so.

Subjective experience and adherence

Patients frequently complain of non-specific subjective effects of medication, saying that they feel 'drugged up' or 'like a zombie'. Complaints about adverse subjective effects, such as the blunting of mood and emotions, slowing down of the thinking process and loss of spontaneity, are well known at the beginning of treatment with psychotropic medicines and these patients consistently complain that medication is making them worse instead of better. A number of studies have investigated the relationship between subjective well-being and adherence to medication; overall there is evidence to support a relationship (Caine and Polinsky, 1979; Van Putten et al., 1980; Naber, 1995), although further research is required. In contrast, the relationship between attitudes towards treatment and adherence has been widely reported in treatment in general and mental health in particular.

Attitudes towards medication and adherence

Case study

Mark is a 23-year-old university student who was admitted to a ward because he believed he could not cope with coursework. He became increasingly isolated at university and expressed suicidal ideas. He was prescribed antidepressants by his doctor, but he refuses to take them for fear of becoming dependent on medication. He was, however, prepared to see a psychologist to talk about his problems.

The case of Mark illustrates a common attitude towards medication. He is reluctant to take prescribed medication, but nevertheless acknowledges that he needs treatment. For this reason, he is prepared to see a psychologist. Whether or not someone takes medication depends very much on their attitude towards it.

A patient's attitude towards treatment is an important factor in medication adherence and one that is influenced by a number of factors (see the earlier sections on health beliefs and health-seeking behaviour). There is abundant evidence to support a relationship between adherence and attitudes towards medication. In the area of psychosis, one of the earliest studies to find such a relationship was by Van Putten et al. (1976), who examined the reactions of 29 patients who habitually refused medication and 30 patients who readily took medication. They found that those patients who refused medication experienced an **ego-syntonic** grandiose psychosis after they discontinued medication. The habitual compliers, in contrast, developed **decompensation**, characterised by effects such as depression and anxiety. This finding has been confirmed by at least 20 studies that have examined a link between adherence and attitudes towards medication. Among these is a study by Loffler et al. (2003), who examined attitudes towards medication to assess the reasons why patients were adherent or non-adherent. Those who were non-adherent expressed negative attitudes towards medication. An important finding was that there was no difference in attitudes to medication between those taking conventional or atypical antipsychotics. Another factor that has been widely implicated in medication adherence is the role of the therapeutic relationship or alliance.

The therapeutic alliance and adherence

It is generally accepted that the communication between the mental health nurse and patient contributes to the welfare of the patients in every aspect of the illness. Patients regard nurses and doctors as respected and trusted sources of health information and this suggests that the health advice offered by a nurse or doctor may have a greater impact than that provided by other sources. Also, patients with mental health problems can be influenced by the attitudes of their treating clinicians and this can affect whether they take medication or not. Despite this widely accepted view, it was not until recently that the role of the therapeutic relationship in outcome and recovery has been systematically examined.

There is indirect evidence to suggest that a positive relationship with the mental health nurse is essential in improving medication adherence (Frank and Gunderson, 1990; Olfson et al., 2000). A patient's perception of the mental health nurse's interest in them, and how the nurse explained the reasons for taking medication and its side effects, all seem to be crucial in improving a positive therapeutic relationship. A strong therapeutic relationship based on trust, clear information, and reinforcement via educational programmes using patients' coffee groups have been shown to improve adherence, according to findings by Dorevitch et al. (1993) and Frank and Gunderson (1990).

Alternatively, Weiden et al. (1986) suggested that there are **counter-transference** issues that can make non-adherence worse. They stated that health professionals frequently see patients as hopeless and incurable and they develop an indifferent attitude towards such patients. They also asserted that another counter-transference issue is when a nurse refuses to empathise with a patient's reasons for non-adherence and, therefore, the patient develops an oppositional behaviour that is detrimental to future collaboration with treatment.

In summary, the therapeutic alliance between practitioner and patient is an important factor in medication adherence and we will return to this topic later in the chapter. There is also sufficient evidence to support the view that adherence is influenced by socio-environmental factors.

Socio-environmental factors

The more support people get from family and friends or significant others, the better the outcome in any health intervention. The evidence shows that patients living with family members are likely to be more adherent to medication and this is particularly true for those suffering from psychotic illnesses (Olfson et al., 2000). As early as 1984, Caton et al. noted that involving families in planning the discharge of patients from hospital can improve adherence and treatment outcome. This was supported by a study by Olfson et al. (2000), who found that patients with families who refuse to become involved in their care were at high risk of non-adherence to antipsychotics.

In a study that examined the role of **expressed emotion** on treatment outcome Sellwood et al. (2003) found that, if patients lived with carers with high levels of expressed emotion, they were three times more likely to be non-adherent to medication than if they lived separately. This finding is supported by a more recent study by Marom and colleagues (2005), who found that critical comments were associated with earlier first and second readmissions compared with low critical comments.

In summary, there is ample evidence to show that negative socio-environmental factors impact negatively on medication adherence. Similarly, the use of **psychoactive** substances, such as cannabis, is known to retard recovery because it makes a patient's non-adherence to medication worse. But before we can discuss the role of psychoactive substances, please try Activity 3.5.

Activity 3.5   *Critical thinking*

Jane is a 35-year-old single woman who lives with her two young children on the sixth floor of a high-rise building owned by the council. As she can't often go out in the evenings, her social life is restricted, and there are no family members living nearby. She has suffered from depression since her first child was born and she is prescribed antidepressants. She accepts that the medication helps, but she finds it difficult to be fully adherent to her treatment.

• What factors impede Jane from being fully adherent to her medication?

An outline answer is provided at the end of the chapter.

Substance misuse and adherence to medication

You will have come across patients suffering from a mental health problem who also use illicit drugs or alcohol. These patients are commonly referred to as suffering from a **dual diagnosis** or **co-**

morbid substance misuse. Previous research has consistently established that patients with dual diagnosis are less likely to adhere to medication (Scher-Svanum et al., 2006). An earlier study by Kashner et al. (1991) discovered that patients who abused substances were 13 times more likely to be non-adherent to medication than those who did not. More recently, Olfson et al. (2000) found that those patients who misused substances were at greater risk of non-adherence to medication than those who did not abuse substances after discharge from hospital. Overall, there is accumulating evidence supporting the role of psychoactive substances in medication adherence.

However, even if factors that pertain to adherence are improved, some patients do not get the full benefit of medication because of its limited efficacy, for a variety of reasons.

Benefits and limitations of medication

Despite the effectiveness of medication in assisting people with mental health problems, you will come across patients who fail to respond to these medicines. This is because, despite evidence of efficacy, most patients show an **idiosyncratic response** to psychotropic medication. In other words, while a particular medication might be effective in one individual, the same medicine and dosage could be totally ineffective in a second person or cause severe adverse effects in a third person. Considering this situation, when is non-adherence with medication a problem? Weiden et al. (1997) have suggested that non-adherence to medication is a problem only when treatment is effective. A necessary step towards understanding non-adherence behaviour is first to understand medication effectiveness.

If we consider the efficacy of antipsychotic medicines, for example, we find that most patients continue to have symptoms despite being on medication, and many others will relapse even if they are taking medication. In addition, it is well known that some psychotropic medication causes adverse side effects such as Parkinsonism, akathisia and dystonia (see sections on these on pages 145–7). Patients who have these side effects are less likely to be adherent, which in turn compromises outcome. The newer generation of antipsychotic medicines, such as olanzapine, have a reduced neurological side-effects profile, but they can cause other problems such as weight gain and sexual dysfunction. The older or classical antidepressants, such as the **tricyclics**, have adverse side effects such as **sedation** and **cardiotoxicity** and can induce movement disorders. The newer antidepressants, the SSRIs (selective serotonin reuptake inhibitors) can cause sleep disturbance and sexual dysfunction. The problem of poor effectiveness of medication also occurs for those taking antidepressants and anti-anxiety medication. Therefore, even if patients are adherent to medication, some are disappointed by the lack of its efficacy. So it may not be fair to call someone non-adherent when they are only gaining modest benefit from medication. In cases where patients find medication helpful, nurses need strategies for improving adherence. To enable you to work effectively with patients, you need to develop a therapeutic alliance.

The therapeutic alliance

In the classical medical relationship, the person receiving the help is the patient but the person making the decisions is the doctor. The patient is then expected to comply with the doctor's orders as a passive recipient of help. Further, the doctor decides who is sick by providing them with a sick certificate; in turn, the sick person is expected to adopt a sick role. Unfortunately, this paternalistic approach is fraught with problems. Also, the growth of consumerism has meant that patients are increasingly taking an active part in their treatment. More importantly, there is research evidence suggesting that people who play an active role in their treatment are more likely to recover a lot quicker than those who play a passive role (see page 62 earlier in the chapter). As a mental health nurse, the need to establish a therapeutic relationship or alliance is a basic tenet of your practice. It is an essential tool that facilitates effective care. So what is a therapeutic alliance?

The therapeutic alliance has been described as a patient's capacity to collaborate productively with the therapist because the therapist is perceived as a helping professional with good intentions. In other words, it is generally viewed as involving an agreement between therapist and patient on the goals of treatment, the tasks needed to accomplish those goals, and a sense of a personal bond between therapist and patient.

The therapeutic alliance has been discussed in the psychotherapy literature for nearly a century and, historically, it was the first concept to be developed in order to capture the special role performed by the patient–psychotherapist relationship. In 1912, Freud outlined the first references to the therapeutic alliance by highlighting its importance as a vehicle for success in psychoanalysis. Some authors have even stated that the quality of the therapeutic alliance is more important than the type of psychotherapy in predicting positive therapeutic outcomes (Safran et al., 2011). In a landmark **empirical study**, the therapeutic alliance was found to have the same effect on outcome regardless of whether the treatment was psychotherapy or **pharmacotherapy**. In another study, Krupnick et al. (1996) examined 225 individuals with depression having outpatient treatment and either interpersonal psychotherapy, cognitive behavioural therapy (CBT), medication with clinical management, or a placebo with clinical management. The study found that the quality of the therapeutic alliance accounted for most of the variance in treatment outcome, regardless of the kind of therapy. As a result, it has been suggested that the therapeutic alliance is a prerequisite for all therapies.

In terms of medication adherence, there is evidence that a relatively strong therapeutic alliance during the opening phase of treatment may be the best predictor of good outcome. An important study that underscored this was by Marder et al. (1983), who found that patients with schizophrenia who were adherent to prescribed medications were more likely to be satisfied with their physicians, to feel their physicians understood them and to feel their treating physicians had their best interests at heart.

Developing a therapeutic alliance

As a nurse, you should help to foster a positive alliance with the patient by identifying with their treatment goals and you should also identify with the healthy aspects of the patient's self that is striving to reach those goals. A patient will then experience their therapists as collaborators who are working with them rather than against them. Developing a good alliance with patients will require you not only to be positive and empathetic, but also to work within a collaborative framework – a partnership in which the patient sees themselves as a respected participant.

A good example of how to foster a therapeutic relationship is provided by Gabbard (2005), who noted that *The therapeutic alliance may be the most essential element of adherence . . .* (pp108–9). You should collaborate with your patient to identify mutually agreed treatment goals and strategies, including medications, and view your patient as a key stakeholder in the treatment-planning process. The focus of adherence should be on shared decision-making between the patient and the nurse in order to determine the most appropriate treatment approach. The nurse listens to the patient with empathy in order to build a strong relationship with the patient. This involves identifying patient concerns regarding medications and addressing any barriers to adherence that are identified in order to establish a strong nurse–patient therapeutic alliance. At the same time, as a nurse, you need to be aware of your own feelings that may arise in dealing with the non-adherent patient. Patients and nurses do not often agree on risk factors for non-adherence. By discussing patients' perceptions regarding medications, nurses have the opportunity to address patient concerns without assuming they already know the barriers that may be contributing to adherence problems in a specific patient.

In people with schizophrenia, establishing rapport with the patient can be challenging. However, a therapeutic alliance with a patient increases the likelihood of the patient staying in therapy, adhering to prescribed medications and achieving a better outcome. In his discussion of the therapeutic alliance, Gabbard (2005) noted that mental health professionals ought to be innovative and find some common ground with patients such as music, films, holiday places and sports. This allows the patient and nurse to share common interests and provides an opportunity for the therapeutic relationship to grow. If the patient expresses delusions, you should not challenge these but should view them as metaphors that can provide insights into the patient's inner conflicts.

You should further help to foster the alliance by focusing on a patient's strengths and accept without judgement bizarre behaviour, feelings and thoughts that others do not understand. As the alliance develops, you should work with the patient to identify specific relapse triggers in order to assist the patient in relapse prevention.

As noted above, engaging patients with schizophrenia in a therapeutic alliance can be difficult. The process can take up to six months, and you should not become pessimistic if the patient is not engaged in a collaborative therapeutic relationship after several months. Based on the results discussed by Frank and Gunderson (1990), if an alliance has not formed after six months, a re-evaluation of the therapy may be warranted.

In establishing a therapeutic alliance with a depressed patient, the nurse should simply listen and empathise with the patient's point of view, while attempting to gain a better comprehension of the patient's understanding of the illness. You should empathise with the painfulness of the depression and enlist the patient's help in a collaborative search for the underlying causes. You should avoid passing 'cheerleading' comments such as 'you have so much to live for'. These comments are often understood to be a lack of empathy and can lead to the patient feeling worse and not understood. Also, you should avoid interpreting a patient's behaviour or mood. Typical statements such as 'You are not really depressed – you're angry' should be avoided, as this may be understood as a lack of empathy on your part. In addition to developing a sound therapeutic alliance with your patient, you need to have an understanding of strategies that have been employed to improve adherence.

Strategies for improving adherence to medication

There is growing acceptance that medication non-adherence is a significant problem that affects recovery and outcome in people with mental health issues. Despite this, there is a limited evidence base for the use of interventions that target the specific factors causing non-adherence. This is due in part to the complex multi-factorial nature of the concept of adherence. Also, the measurement of adherence has proved to be problematic (see pages 60–1 earlier in this chapter). However, interventions such as psychotherapy have proved to be successful in alleviating poor medication adherence.

Several intervention strategies can be used, such as alliance building, motivational interviewing, psychoeducation, psychotherapy and/or CBT, and these will be briefly reviewed later. It is important for you also to assess your patients' motivation or readiness to change behaviour.

Psychotherapy

Psychological counselling may produce an emotional improvement that can increase the desire and ability of some patients to improve self-care. This is particularly so for those who are depressed and there is some evidence to support the use of psychotherapy to improve medication adherence. It is assumed that, by coming to understand their treatment rights and responsibilities, patients can break the cycle. Improvements in feelings of self-worth and independence may then produce positive behavioural outcomes, which may include improved adherence. Thus, addressing depression using psychotherapy appears to be a logical approach for some non-adherent patients.

Psychoeducation

Psychoeducation is a specific form of education that is aimed at helping people with mental health problems to access the facts about a broad range of mental illnesses in a clear and concise manner. It is also a way of accessing and learning strategies to deal with mental illness and its effects. It has remained consistently popular as a tool for families and carers to be able to make sense of what is happening to a person who is experiencing a mental illness and to help them to care for that person. With regard to improving medication adherence, psychoeducation has been the mainstay intervention. Many of these strategies involve individual or group counselling sessions and/or use of written and audiovisual materials on diagnoses, medications and side effects. For maximum benefit, psychoeducation should be used in conjunction with other therapies.

Cognitive behavioural therapy

Cognitive behavioural therapy (CBT) is a form of psychotherapy that emphasises the importance of finding new ways of thinking and behaving to deal with current problems. In a cognitive approach, adherence is conceptualised as a coping behaviour based on an individual's perception of the illness and his or her beliefs about medications. Hence interventions based on CBT seek to assist the patient to question his/her automatic thoughts regarding their medications. The emphasis on CBT is to help the patient mentally link medication adherence to symptom reduction and personal health. The nurse should follow a programme manual and have several individual sessions with patients.

CBT has been demonstrated to improve adherence among patients with serious mental illness and to increase insight in patients with schizophrenia. Other behavioural approaches to improve adherence include conditioning, rewards, cues, reminders and skills training. These interventions seek to promote, modify and reinforce behaviours related to adherence in patients, including those with psychotic disorders. More recently, motivational interviewing principles have been added to CBT approaches to enhance adherence.

Motivational interviewing

Motivational interviewing (MI) is a directive, client-centred counselling style for eliciting behaviour change by helping clients to explore and resolve **ambivalence**. The examination and resolution of ambivalence is its central purpose, and the counsellor is intentionally directive in pursuing this goal. It has been used in many areas of health, such as treating addictions, and is now being applied to patients with other mental health problems to assess a patients' level of motivation towards adopting medication-adherent behaviours.

Change, as conceptualised in MI, can be viewed as a process with multiple stages, with the initial stage being *pre-contemplation* and the last stage being *action maintenance*. In using MI, you should adapt the intervention to the patient's current position on the change cycle. Basic principles of MI include expressing empathy for patients, supporting self-efficacy in an unwavering manner, highlighting discrepancies between the patient's current health behaviours and core values, and rolling with resistance.

'Rolling with resistance' means that you should not challenge the patient's resistance to medications, but rather explore the resistance in order to understand the patient's perspective. The patient may then be better able to identify their own solutions to potential barriers to medication adherence. In this approach, self-efficacy is defined as patients' confidence in their ability to adopt healthy behaviour changes, such as adhering to prescribed medications, which nurses support and enhance by communicating their belief in patients' ability to make these changes.

Highlighting discrepancies involves identifying patients' priorities and goals, and making connections between adhering to medications and attaining those goals. MI principles conceptualise 'resistance' as occurring when the nurse's level of intervention is inappropriate for the patient's stage of change or perception of the issue. Resistance is viewed as a measure of the therapeutic alliance (see pages 71–2). In an MI approach, you do not confront the patient about the need for change, but rather you encourage a discussion about the pros and cons of making a change. When patients verbalise the positive aspects of change on their own, they are more likely to adopt the change. MI sessions employ four major technical approaches during the intervention, which can be summarised by the acronym OARS.

- Ask **O**pen-ended questions.
- **A**ffirm patients' self-efficacy.
- **R**eflect on patients' thoughts via active listening.
- **S**ummarise patients' narratives to help resolve ambivalence and promote change.

As mentioned earlier, using MI in combination with cognitive approaches has been reported to significantly improve adherence in patients with a dual diagnosis of depression and cocaine dependence, as well as in patients with psychosis. This integrated approach has sometimes been referred to as a concordance process.

Concordance-based approach to adherence

'Medication concordance' is a term used to signify that the health professional and patient have come to a shared agreement about therapeutic goals. To be able to reach a therapeutic goal, the nurse will have to develop a rapport with the patient, understand the problem from the patient's point of view, come to a shared understanding and agreement about the problem, imparted information about the proposed treatment, and give alternative choices. Medication concordance utilises the therapeutic alliance and shared decision-making process as its cornerstone and requires a deeper understanding of patients' health beliefs. Such an approach is likely to promote medication adherence.

Collaboratively address risk factors for non-adherence

Risk factors associated with non-adherence were discussed earlier (see pages 66–9) and it is important for you to be aware of and identify these potential barriers early in the treatment process. Unfortunately, one of main disadvantages of current intervention strategies to improve adherence is that they are not designed to target specific risk factors, and further research is necessary in this area. However, the goal of recognising risk factors for medication non-adherence is for you to identify individuals at high risk of non-adherence and allocate time to spend with the patient to address medication issues.

During the first interview, you should explore the patient's expectations in order to help them to accept treatment that is in some way consistent with their expectations. You can initiate a discussion of adherence by asking the patient directly 'Is there anything that is preventing you from taking your medication?' At all times, you should avoid taking an authoritarian approach, as this may backfire, leading to the patient being non-adherent. You should provide education to the patient about the reasons for recommending particular types of medicines and discuss potential side effects. But you should always ask if the patient is happy for you to give unsolicited advice, as some patients may object. This type of approach is likely to have a positive impact on the therapeutic alliance and minimises resistance. Patients and mental health professionals sometimes differ in their opinions regarding the value of various medication selection factors. Therefore, you need to promote an open discussion about medication and the decision-making process in order to increase the likelihood that the patient will adhere to prescribed medications. More importantly, it is essential that you assess the patient's level of motivation to change behaviour.

Assess readiness to change behaviour

It is critical for you to assess the patient's motivation to adopt a particular treatment recommendation and likelihood of being adherent to medication. If you begin by discussing psychoeducational information about medications without assessing a patient's motivation to change, the unmotivated patient is less likely to initiate and maintain recommended treatment. Unfortunately, most patients do not come forward and say 'I want to change my behaviour.' This will require motivation and therefore it is important for you to understand the theory under-pinning motivation to change behaviour. The theoretical model widely used to assess motivation to change was formulated by Prochaska and DiClemente (1984a) and is called the stages of behaviour change (or transtheoretical) model (see Figure 3.2).

The transtheoretical model in health psychology assesses an individual's readiness to act on new, healthier behaviour, and provides processes, taken over a period, to guide the individual through the stages of change to action and maintenance (see Figure 3.2).

Patients in the *pre-contemplation stage* may not believe that medication adherence is important and may not have any desire to change. Those patients in the *contemplation stage* are thinking of changing but are not yet fully dedicated to changing. These patients are more aware that non-adherence can be problematic to their health. Patients in the *preparation stage* are intending to adhere to their medications regularly, but may have several barriers preventing them from doing so. Patients who are *taking action* are actively working to take their medications regularly, while patients in the *maintenance stage* are doing so on a consistent basis.

In deciding to change a current behaviour, patients must balance the pros and cons of the change (decisional balance) according to their lifestyles and health beliefs. As patients move from unawareness of any problem, through contemplating a change, to actually carrying out the action, the pros increase and the cons decrease. Once the change has been accomplished, self-efficacy – the confidence to overcome difficulties and maintain the new behaviour pattern – is important (Julius et al., 2009).

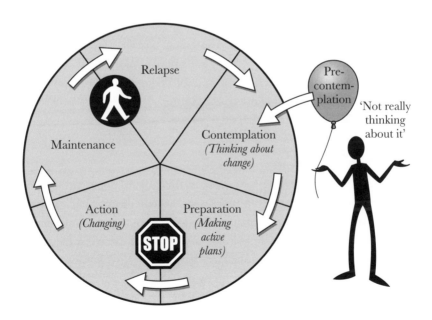

Figure 3.2: Stages of behaviour change model

You will need to reinforce any progress and encourage the patient during the entire process of change. In the early stages, emotional and cognitive factors are important to raise consciousness and increase motivation to take the first step. In the later stages, there is more emphasis on commitment, action and avoiding relapse; defining goals and teaching medication administration skills and relapse-prevention strategies become more important. Motivation and supplying relevant information therefore need to be geared specifically to the patient's stage of readiness to change; however, you should take care not to pressure the patient as this may lead to resistance. Table 3.1 integrates the transtheoretical model and basic intervention strategies to improve adherence with medication.

In assessing motivation and readiness to change, you could start by agreeing on an agenda with your patient to address medication adherence and related issues, including the following suggested by Borrelli et al. (2007).

*   'I'd like to take some time to discuss your medication.' 'How many times this past week did you take your medication?'
*   'How does taking your medication fit into your daily routine?'
*   'On a scale of 1 to 10, how motivated are you to take your medication?'
*   'What do you think it would take to make you a 10 on this scale as opposed to where you are now?'
*   'What do you feel is preventing you from taking your medications as prescribed?'
*   'What are the positive/negative aspects of taking your medications?'
*   'How would taking your medications regularly change your life?'
*   'How would taking your medications regularly help you?'

You should encourage your patient to discuss the positive and negative aspects of taking medication as prescribed. The patient should be prompted to verbalise their own intent to change in order to increase the likelihood that they will adopt the behaviours necessary for change. You should use reflective listening skills and, after the patient has verbalised their thoughts, summarise the pros of taking the prescribed medications to the patient in their own words. You should help the patient make associations between the benefits of taking medication and symptom reduction (Julius et al., 2009). Finally, when patients do make steps towards behaviour change, you should give positive feedback to reinforce these behaviours.

Carer involvement

As discussed previously, families can have an impact on patients' adherence to prescribed medications. Family members with negative attitudes regarding medications and other misconceptions about the nature of their loved one's mental illness can be a barrier to adherence to prescribed medications (Julius et al., 2009). Studies have demonstrated improved adherence and reductions in relapse in patients whose family members are actively engaged in their treatment and receive some level of intervention from mental health professionals. Family members should be involved in treatment planning and addressing potential concerns about recommended treatment. You should ensure that relatives are involved in providing educational information to the patient about the diagnosis and treatment. It is also important to identify and discuss the family's ability and willingness to support the patient and encourage adherence to recommended treatments. You

Stage of change	Process in operation/ explanation	Patient characteristics	Possible intervention
Stage one Precontemplation	1. Consciousness raising 2. Social liberation	1. Rebellion 2. Resignation 3. Rationalisation 4. Reluctance 5. Reinforce progress	1. Provide choices 2. Build hope 3. Encourage reflection 4. Give information
Stage two Contemplation	1. Consciousness raising 2. Social liberation 3. Emotional arousal 4. Self-evaluation 5. Commitment	1. Open to information 2. Ambivalence	1. Provide information 2. Help to weigh pros and cons 3. Increase self-efficacy 4. Reinforce progress
Stage three Preparation	1. Social liberation 2. Emotional arousal 3. Self-re-evaluation	Determination	1. Help set goals 2. Provide strategies for change 3. Reinforce progress
Stage four Action	1. Social liberation 2. Commitment 3. Reward 4. Environmental control 5. Helping relationships	1. Actively changing 2. Self-evaluation	1. Teach skills and self-management 2. Guide attribution process 3. Reinforce progress
Stage five Maintenance	1. Commitment 2. Reward 3. Countering 4. Environmental control 5. Helping relationships	1. At risk/relapse 2. Self-evaluation	1. Teach relapse prevention strategies 2. Encourage continuation 3. Reinforce progress

Table 3.1: Stages of change and associated patient characteristics and possible interventions (from Chapman et al., 2000).

should provide emotional support to families to enable them to cope with the mental illness of their loved one. For example, you might encourage family members to participate in local support groups, such as those sponsored by voluntary organisations (Julius et al., 2009).

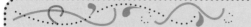

Chapter summary

Current methods of treating and aiding recovery in people with mental health problems place special emphasis on establishing a shared decision-making approach where patients take an active part in their treatment and this necessitates building a therapeutic alliance.

Despite potential benefits derived from taking medication, people with mental health problems sometimes do not take medication and this can have enormous personal, social and economic consequences in their lives. The reasons for poor adherence are many and diverse but include adverse side effects, attitudes to treatment and severity of illness. Because of the importance of medication adherence, several strategies have been devised to improve it. One of the more popular strategies uses a combination of CBT, psycho-education and MI principles to treat mental problems. Patient involvement and establishing a good therapeutic alliance are central to the recovery model of care.

Activities: brief outline answers

Activity 3.1 Partial adherence (page 61)

Some reasons why patients are partially adherent include: they may not consider themselves to be ill; lack family support; adverse side effects; or they believe that their illness could be treated by other means instead of medication. A poor relationship with the mental health professional can impact on adherence.

Activity 3.2 Julio's health belief system (page 63)

Julio's view of his illness is not invalid at all if his own cultural background is considered. People's health belief systems are in part shaped by their culture. More importantly, Julio accepts that something is not right, but it is the explanation he offers that is shaped by his culture and he therefore seeks a culturally appropriate remedy.

Activity 3.3 Barriers to seeking treatment (page 65)

There are many barriers to seeking help. The most common tend be lack of understanding regarding the illness, financial constraints, language, cultural differences between the patient and provider in the interpretation of symptoms, and inappropriate services that do not reflect the needs of the people they serve.

Activity 3.4 Insight into illness (page 67)

Some of the factors that may lead someone to think they have no mental health problems, despite evidence to the contrary, include severity of the illness, social isolation and cultural beliefs.

Activity 3.5 Medication adherence (page 70)

Reasons that may impede Jane from benefiting fully from medication include environmental factors – she lives on the sixth floor of a high-rise flat, which is hardly ideal for someone with two young children. Also, it appears she has little support from family and friends and this contributes towards poor adherence.

Further reading

Amador, XF and David, A (2004) *Insight and Psychosis: Awareness of illness in schizophrenia and related disorders.* Oxford: Oxford University Press.

A valuable book that details awareness of illness and how it is a barrier to seeking health.

Blackwell, B (1998) From compliance to alliance: a quarter century of research, in Blackwell, B (ed.) *Treatment Compliance and the Therapeutic Alliance.* Amsterdam: Harwood Academic, pp1–15.

A very useful book that comprehensively covers factors that affect medication adherence in serious mental illness. The chapter by Cohen on treatment compliance in schizophrenia explains adherence from a public health viewpoint.

Miller, WR and Rollick, S (1991) *Motivational Interviewing: Preparing people to change.* New York: Guilford Press.

A very useful book that deals with motivational interviewing.

Useful websites

www.adultmeducation.com

This website deals specifically with adherence issues for older adults and provides information on different adherence strategies.

www.babcp.com

The BABCP is the leading organisation for the theory, practice and development of CBT in the UK. It has over 8,000 members including nurses, trainees, counsellors, psychologists and psychiatrists.

Chapter 4
Essential anatomy and physiology of the brain

NMC Standards for Pre-registration Nursing Education

This chapter will address the following competencies:

Domain 3: Nursing practice and decision-making

2. All nurses must possess a broad knowledge of the structure and functions of the human body, and other relevant knowledge from the life, behavioural and social sciences as applied to health, ill health, disability, ageing and death. They must have an in-depth knowledge of common physical and mental health problems and treatments in their own field of practice, including co-morbidity and physiological and psychological vulnerability.

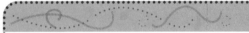

NMC Essential Skills Clusters

This chapter will address the following ESCs:

Cluster: Medicines management

36. People can trust the newly registered graduate nurse to ensure safe and effective practice in medicines management through comprehensive knowledge of medicines, their actions, risks and benefits.

40. People can trust a newly registered graduate nurse to work in partnership with people receiving medical treatments and their carers.

Chapter aims

By the end of this chapter, you should be familiar with:

*   regions of the brain and their functions;
*   specific brain regions that play a part in neural communication;
*   the limbic system and its function;
*   neural networks, neural migration and connectivity;
*   the structure of the neuron;
*   classical neurotransmitters, their function and chemical neurotransmission;
*   the importance of synapses.

Introduction

The human brain is the result of at least four billion years' evolution and is the most complex object known; it is an electrical and chemical powerhouse that sends messages where needed in a perfectly targeted way. The brain weighs about one and half kilograms, and is soft and grey. It is not only where we experience and manipulate the world, but is also responsible for control of our breathing, body temperature, blood pressure and hormones. The brain has no moving parts as do the heart or lungs, and it does not make anything, unlike the kidney, liver or spleen. Unlike the skin or bones, the brain serves no *obvious* purpose, yet we know it is responsible for thoughts, emotions and free will. In short, the simple view of the brain as the most fundamental of all organs may seem rather obvious, but how did we come to such a conclusion? To answer this question, we need to go back in the past and find out what people before us believed about the brain.

In ancient Egypt, the brain was regarded to be a form of 'cranial stuffing' of sorts that served no useful purpose. The heart was instead thought of as the seat of intelligence. This belief is best exemplified by the way ancient Egyptians prepared bodies for mummification, by taking great care in the preparation of organs such as the heart, lungs, liver and stomach, while the brain was simply scooped from the skull. As much as we now know that the brain is the seat of intelligence, colloquial expressions such as 'learning something by heart' or 'suffering from heartache' remain commonly used to this day (Gibb, 2007).

Around 450 BC, the Greek physician Alcmaeon was among the first to recognise the brain's importance, but his view was not universally accepted. A hundred years later, Aristotle reasserted the importance of the heart and suggested that the brain was little more than a cooling system for the heart.

From the first century BC, the prevailing view was that of Galen, a Greek physician who suggested that the heart controlled the four humours: blood, phlegm, yellow bile and black bile. This theory was untrue, of course, but Galen did manage to recognise the link between the brain and memory, emotion and processing of senses. It was not until the 1800s that progress regarding brain physiology was made.

Thomas Willis (1621–75), an English neurologist, was largely credited with advancing knowledge about the brain, being the first person to examine the brain with real scientific rigour. After years of research, he published his ground-breaking *Cerebri Anatome*, providing the first complete description of the brain's regions. He correctly linked memory and higher function with the cerebral hemispheres and he also laid down the basis of brain science terminology. Another breakthrough by Willis correctly proposed that the liquid-filled spaces deep inside the brain, the ventricles, served no significant purpose, whereas before many thought they were the centre of high brain function. Several other scientists contributed to our knowledge of the brain, including Emanuel Swedenborg (1688–1772), Franz Joseph Gall (1758–1828), Paul Pierre Broca (1824–80) and Carl Wernicke (1848–1905). Most importantly, Santiago Ramón y Cajal (1852–1934) published a textbook regarded by many as one of the greatest scientific texts – *Manual of Normal Histology and Micrographic Technique*. He was the first to suggest that the brain and nervous system consisted of discrete cells called the neurons. He described the nervous system and the brain with unparalleled clarity and for his work he received the Nobel Prize for Physiology or Medicine in 1906. These breakthroughs inspired many surgical techniques and drugs discoveries that remedy brain dysfunctions. But the greatest advance of all was that of observing the activity of the living brain.

Brain scanning

Our knowledge of the brain has been greatly enhanced by scanning techniques. The first major attempts at scanning the human brain were by Hans Berger in 1924. He used an electroencephalogram (EEG) to measure human brainwaves and this laid the groundwork for future research into computerised axial tomography (CAT or CT) and positron emission tomography (PET). CAT scans use powerful computers to covert two-dimensional X-ray pictures into three-dimensional images for further study. PET scans use a radioactive 'tracer' substance that is injected directly into the human body. This substance gradually accumulates inside the major organs, at the same time emitting positron radiation, which is detected by a sensor. A more recent and non-invasive technique is functional magnetic resonance imaging (fMRI). This employs the use of a magnet weighing several tons. It relies on the metal-charged ions in our body, including iron. The magnetic properties of the metal charges, such as iron, change in the presence of oxygen. A change in oxygen concentration reflects brain activity and this information is processed by a powerful computer to construct a two- or three-dimensional image of brain activity. This technique allows us to observe the global behaviour of the brain during different types of activities, such as mental arithmetic, reading a book or watching a movie.

In summary, it has taken us centuries to understand even the basic functions of the human brain. Although there is still much we do not know about the brain, we now have a good knowledge of the basic anatomy and physiology of each region of the brain.

Brain regions

In neuroscience, the brain is considered to have at least six main regions: the cerebral hemispheres, diencephalon (thalamus and hypothalamus), midbrain, cerebellum, pons and medulla oblongata. Each brain region in turn has a complex internal structure.

The brainstem

This is the stalk-like part of the brain connecting to the spinal cord and the forebrain, and it is made up of the *pons*, the *medulla oblongata* and the *midbrain* (see Figure 4.1). The brainstem functions as an important relay station for every nerve impulse that passes between the brain and the spinal cord to allow the body to function normally. The medulla oblongata is involved with the control of the unconscious or autonomic part of body function such as blood circulation and muscle tone.

The pons part of the brainstem is situated between the midbrain and the medulla oblongata. The pons's function is to relay signals from the cortex to assist in the control of movement and it is also involved in the control of sleep and arousal. The midbrain is positioned between the hindbrain and the forebrain. The midbrain forms part of the brainstem and connects the brainstem to the forebrain. It is responsible for controlling sensory processes. Before you read further, you need to undertake Activity 4.1.

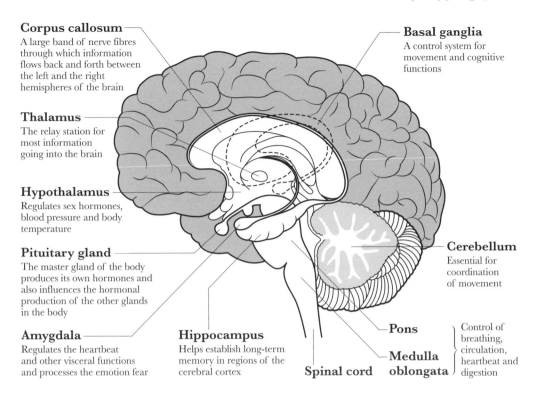

Corpus callosum
A large band of nerve fibres through which information flows back and forth between the left and the right hemispheres of the brain

Thalamus
The relay station for most information going into the brain

Hypothalamus
Regulates sex hormones, blood pressure and body temperature

Pituitary gland
The master gland of the body produces its own hormones and also influences the hormonal production of the other glands in the body

Amygdala
Regulates the heartbeat and other visceral functions and processes the emotion fear

Hippocampus
Helps establish long-term memory in regions of the cerebral cortex

Spinal cord

Basal ganglia
A control system for movement and cognitive functions

Cerebellum
Essential for coordination of movement

Pons

Medulla oblongata
Control of breathing, circulation, heartbeat and digestion

Figure 4.1: A cross-section of the brain showing the major regions and their functions

---

Activity 4.1   *Critical thinking*

If someone is pronounced to be 'clinically dead', what part of the brain plays an important part in coming to this conclusion, and why?

An outline answer is provided at the end of the chapter.

The cerebellum

The cerebellum, or 'little brain', is found behind the brainstem, to which it is connected. It is split into two hemispheres and it has a convoluted surface that makes it look somewhat like a giant walnut (see Figure 4.1). It is one of the earliest brain regions to evolve and the human version is comparatively similar to that of other mammals. As motor systems of mammals became more sophisticated, there was a need to coordinate increasingly accurate movements such as those of the eye, hands and fingers, and this has resulted in the evolution and enlargement of the cerebellum. This is evident in its structure, in which the central part in the oldest and most primitive and outer part of the lobe is concerned with functions unique to humans. It has strong connections with the motor parts of the cortex. The cerebellum has two lobes but, unlike the motor cortex, it controls movements on the same side of the body as itself. When the cerebellum goes wrong, it results in impaired coordination and this is called *ataxia*. The commonest cause of temporary ataxia is consuming alcohol. Now we need to turn our attention to another part of the brain called the diencephalon.

The diencephalon

The diencephalon or 'interbrain' is located between the cerebral hemispheres and above the midbrain. This region of the brain includes the thalamus, hypothalamus, epithalamus, prethalamus or subthalamus, the pituitary gland and other structures (see Figure 4.1).

The egg-shaped *thalamus* is essential for gating and processing sensory information entering the brain. The only exception to this is that it does not process information from the nose. The thalamus processes information and decides whether it needs to be sent to the cortex for conscious consideration. Also, information from the cerebellum and other areas that are involved in movement is sent to the thalamus for processing. Just below the thalamus is the *hypothalamus*, which controls a multitude of functions.

The hypothalamus is connected to almost every other part of the brain and is essential to motivation, including seeking out pleasurable rewards. It also regulates hormonal release and is involved in any activities relating to **homeostasis**. Another important region of the brain is the limbic system, which we will look at next.

The limbic system

In addition to the structures that make up the diencephalon, there are three further major brain structures buried deep beneath the folds of the cortical hemispheres: the basal ganglia, amygdala and hippocampus (see Figure 4.1). These three structures and others form the limbic system, but we are only concerned with the ones mentioned because of the critical role they play in brain function. The limbic lobe is a complex set of three C-shaped structures containing both grey and white matter. It lies deep within the brain and includes portions of all the lobes of the cerebral hemispheres. It is one of the more primitive parts of the brain. It has a central role in memory, learning, emotion, neuroendocrine function and autonomic activities. Clinical conditions involving the limbic system include epilepsy, congenital syndromes, dementias and various psychiatric disorders, as we will see in later chapters.

Connected to the cortex and thalamus is a swollen structure called the *basal ganglia*, which receive most of their input from the cortex and are responsible for coordination of fine movement. Parkinson's disease provides an excellent example of what happens when the basal ganglia are damaged.

Below the hypothalamus is the structure called the *amygdala*. This term comes from the Greek for 'almond' and is a reference to its size and shape. Despite its relatively small size, the amygdala plays an important part in generating emotional responses such as fear and desire, and it is responsible for the way we relate to the world and those around us.

Close to the amygdala is the *hippocampus*, which takes its name from its seahorse-like shape. It is here in the hippocampus that memories are forged. It is also here that experiences are turned into neural pathways that are then stored for future reference. It is now time for you to consider Activity 4.2 before you proceed further.

The hypothalamus is part of a collection of brain tissues called the diencephalon and it is connected to every part of the brain.

- Can you name three main functions of this very important structure?

An outline answer is provided at the end of the chapter.

The cerebral cortex

The crowning achievement of brain evolution in many respects has to be the cerebral cortex. This is a rippling outer layer that gives the human brain most of its unique powers. The cortex grew a lot during a relatively short time and, to accommodate its growth, it became increasingly folded; it is estimated that the human cortex has an area of about one and half square metres and is four millimetres thick. The grey surface of the cortex is due to a vast network of specialised neurons, six layers of which travel down towards the underlying white matter. In the white matter region, they again form a vast number of connections with other neurons. This vast matrix allows for a swift intercommunication, facilitating our powers of thought. The cortex is not a homogeneous region as it is divided into many areas (Gibb, 2007). First, it is divided into two hemispheres, which are themselves divided by deep grooves into four major areas called 'lobes' – the frontal, parietal, occipital and temporal lobes (see Figure 4.2).

The *frontal lobe* lies directly beneath the forehead and is involved in what is collectively termed 'higher functions'. These higher functions include attention, planning, language and movement. It is like a master control unit that helps to integrate information and govern what the rest of the brain does. Behind the frontal lobe and at the top of the head is the *parietal lobe*, which processes a lot of sensory information, allowing us to perceive the world and our place within it. At the back, the *occipital lobe* deals primarily with vision and it is here that signals from the eyes become

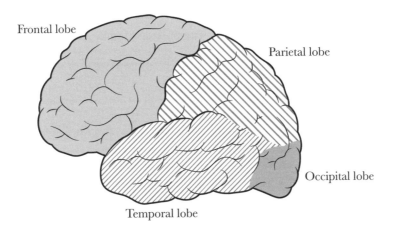

Frontal lobe

Parietal lobe

Occipital lobe

Temporal lobe

Figure 4.2: The four lobes of the cerebral cortex

transformed into useful visual representations. Finally, the *temporal lobes* are located on each side of the brain and they mainly process sound and language. Because they are connected to the hippocampus they are also concerned with memory formation and retrieval.

The corpus callosum

The brain's hemispheres are held together by a bundle of tissues called the *corpus callosum*. This is the largest bundle of nerve fibres in the brain and it is also the main channel through which information flows from one side of the brain to the other. If there is damage to the corpus callosum, this can give rise to illnesses such as epilepsy. Now it is time to turn your attention to Activity 4.3.

| Activity 4.3 | Critical thinking |

The cerebral cortex is a highly evolved part of the brain. Name the sub-regions of the cerebral cortex and their functions.

An outline answer is provided at the end of the chapter.

Part	Function
Frontal lobe	Memory, consciousness, motor activities, judgements, controls emotional response and language
Parietal lobe	For visual attention, touch perception, goal-directed voluntary movements, manipulation of objects and integration of different senses
Occipital lobe	Vision
Temporal lobes	Hearing ability, memory, visual perceptions, object categorisation
Midbrain	Connects brainstem to the forebrain, controls sensory process
Pons	Relays signals from cortex and is involved in sleep arousal
Thalamus	Processes sensory information entering the brain
Hypothalamus	Connected to every part of the brain, important in motivation and seeking reward
Cerebellum	Controls movement
Basal ganglia	Receives information from the cortex, responsible for coordinating fine movements
Amygdala	Generates emotional responses such as fear and desire
Hippocampus	Forges memory, and experiences are converted into neural pathways.

Table 4.1: A summary of parts of the brain and their functions

The neural network

The nervous system, consisting of the brain and the central nervous system (CNS), is made up of specialised cells that communicate with each other and with other cells in the body. These specialised cells are called nerve cells or *neurons* and the human brain consists of billions of them. Each neuron is linked to thousands of other neurons through small spaces called *synapses*. The brain has trillions of these specialised connections. When neurons malfunction, this can result in behavioural symptoms (Stahl, 2008). The malfunction of the neurons can be corrected by medicines that work on these neurons to relieve behavioural symptoms. This section will describe the function of a normal neuron as a way of understanding psychiatric disorder and, as we will see in later chapters, this helps us to understand how psychotropic medicines work.

The structure of the neuron

You will find that, in many textbooks, the neuron is portrayed with a generic structure, but the reality is that many neurons have unique structures. Neurons vary so much in shape that it is not possible to describe a 'typical' one, but they do have three major features in common. Each has a cell body containing a *nucleus* and an extension called the *axon*, which transmits nerve impulses to other cells. The third major feature of neurons is one or more tree-like branching extensions called *dendrites* (see Figure 4.3).

When activated, neurons transmit a wave of electrochemical change, called an *impulse*. The starting point of an impulse could be a sense organ such as the skin, an eye or an ear, or it could be at a dendrite that has received a message from another neuron.

The dendrites collect information and send it to the neuron's control centre which is the *cell body* (see Figure 4.3). The cell body also determines the overall shape and behaviour of the neuron by producing protein in accordance with instructions issued by **DNA**. The cell body pools together the data from each branch of the dendrite to create an overall signal. This signal is then passed to an area known as the *axon hillock* (indicated by the 'axon' arrow in Figure 4.3), which serves as an electrical integrator. It is here at the axon hillock that a decision is made whether or not to fire an electrical impulse in response to incoming electrical information. If the overall charge from the dendrites reaches a particular threshold, a signal will be fired. The axon will propagate

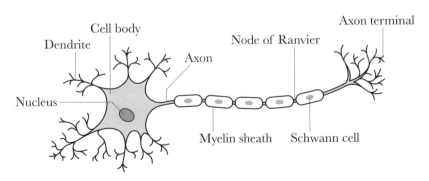

Figure 4.3: Structure of a neuron showing dendrites, cell body axon and myelin sheath

chemical signals within the internal cell matrix, but it will also propagate these electrical signals travelling along the membrane to the presynaptic zone.

The firing of an electrical impulse down an axon is less straightforward than the flow of electrons down a copper wire (Gibb, 2007). Just as in copper wire, which is often insulated with plastic, many axons are insulated with a fatty substance called *myelin sheath*, which reduces the risk of short circuits caused by nearby axons. **Myelin** sheath also helps to speed up electrical impulses, which jump from one node of Ranvier to the next (see Figure 4.3), a process known as *saltory conduction*.

When the electrical impulse reaches the end of the neuron, it causes the activation of the *synaptic vesicles*, which contain chemical substances called *neurotransmitters*. These neurotransmitters amplify or modulate electrical signals being passed to the neighbouring neuron. The action of neuro-transmitters is described in more detail in a later section. Meanwhile, we need to turn our attention to what you have just learned and test your understanding.

Activity 4.4   *Evidence-based practice and research*

Search the internet and find out what illnesses are associated with a dysfunction of the following regions of the brain: frontal lobe, amygdala, hippocampus, pons and substantia nigra.

Answers are provided at the end of the chapter.

Neural development

As previously discussed, the importance of understanding how the brain develops cannot be overstated. It is a necessary step towards understanding how psychotropic medicines work. This section will discuss the basic concepts of neural development. Initially, the section will focus on describing the anatomical basis of neurotransmission before discussing how neurons migrate, form synapses and demonstrate plasticity.

Time course of neural development

The understanding of human neural development is changing at an extremely fast pace thanks largely to stem cell research and advances in forms of brain imaging techniques. The process of neural development starts when the egg fuses with the sperm and a process of cell division (mitosis) commences.

Cells differentiate into immature neurons and those that are selected migrate to different parts of the brain and differentiate into different types of neurons. The formation of new neurons, or *neurogenesis*, continues throughout adult life in some parts of the brain and, in particular, in the hippocampus. The hippocampus is an area that appears to be particularly sensitive to the effects of stress, ageing and disease. Neurogenesis of the hippocampus can be stimulated through learn-ing, psychotherapy, exercise or even certain types of psychotherapy and psychotropic medicines. It is also known that a neuron may fail to develop during childhood, either because of a developmental disease or because of a lack of appropriate neural or environmental stimulation (Stahl, 2008). Part of neural development takes the form of neural migration.

Neural migration

As much as it is surprising that the production of neurons occurs in the mature adult brain, it is also surprising that, periodically, under specified conditions, neurons can kill themselves. This form of suicide is called *apoptosis* and up to 90 per cent of the neurons the brain makes during foetal development commit apoptosis. The reason for apoptosis is that there is an excess of neurons during the prenatal stage of neural development and only a few will be selected for migration. Some of these neurons are healthy and some are defective. In normal brain development, the good neurons are chosen and the defective neurons commit apoptosis. However, if there is a neurodevelopmental disorder, some defective neurons may be chosen for migration and this will cause neurological or psychiatric disorders in later life.

Scenario

A 46-year-old mother with a son suffering from schizophrenia informed a nurse that, while she was seven months pregnant with her son, she contracted a viral infection that lasted three weeks.

Trauma or infection to the mother during pregnancy can have profound effects on the neural development of the unborn child. Viral infection during the third trimester of pregnancy has been robustly linked to schizophrenia (O'Connell et al., 1997). It is possible that viral infection interferes somewhat with neural selection, whereby defective neurons are selected for migration.

As we have previously discussed, not only must the correct neurons be selected, they must also migrate to the right parts of the brain. Incorrect migration of neurons can cause a neurodevelopmental disorder such as epilepsy or attention deficit hyperactive disorder (ADHD). Now we will turn our attention to another process that involves the formation of the synapse, or synaptogenesis.

Synaptogenesis

Once neurons settle down in their respective areas, they form synapses (see Figure 4.4). A synapse is the space between two dendritic neurons. It is a structure that permits a neuron to pass an electrical or chemical signal to another cell.

During normal development, neurons from different parts of the brain are appropriately directed to their target dendrites forming correct synapses. In abnormal development, however, the wrong dendrites will form synapses with the wrong neurons, resulting in incorrect wiring. In later life, this could lead to abnormal information transfer, which affects neural communication and the ability of neurons to function normally. We now turn our attention to the concept of neural plasticity.

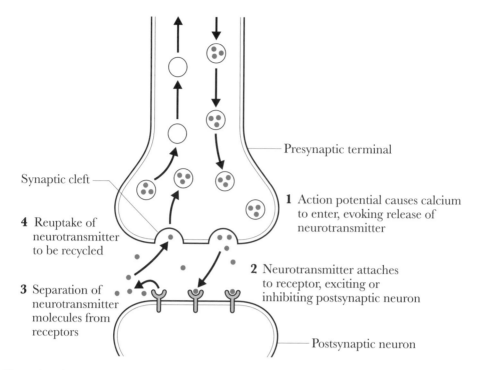

Figure 4.4: A synapse with neurotransmitters

Neural plasticity

The synapses can form on any part of the neuron and not just the dendrites. Synapses that are formed on any part of the neuron other than the dendrites are called asymmetrical. Once a synapse is formed, it remains a dynamic area of intense molecular activity and in many ways a synapse is under constant revision as long as it is functional, with molecular maintenance and alterations constantly instituted to respond to changing conditions (Stahl, 2008). For example, the surface area of the pre- and post-synaptic membrane can increase to accommodate numbers and types of receptors that facilitate communication. Increased neurotransmission may lead to an increased number of post-synaptic receptors, or in some cases whole axons can develop. Also, if the brain stays active, neurons will be preserved and new ones can even form, but if it is inactive, the neural connection will become weak and may be 'pruned off'.

In summary, the dendritic tree of a neuron not only sprouts new branches, grows and establishes a multitude of new synaptic connections throughout its life, but can also remove, alter, trim or destroy such connections when necessary.

Now that you have read about the mechanism of neural plasticity, you need to undertake Activity 4.5 to test your understanding.

Activity 4.5   *Critical thinking*

In a group or as an individual, find out the typical age of onset for psychosis.

• How does this period of onset relate to neural pruning?

An outline answer is provided at the end of the chapter.

Chemical neurotransmission

Neurotransmission can be defined as the passing of signals from nerve cell to nerve cell through chemicals or electric impulses. Chemical neurotransmission constitutes the cornerstone of neuroscientific principles and the concept has been in existence in various forms since early Greek civilisation, but it was not until 1877 that the German physiologist Emil Du Bois-Reymond (1818–96) suggested that there might be substances in the body, electrical in nature, responsible for neurotransmission (Lopez-Munoz and Alamo, 2009). We now call these substances *neurotransmitters*. In 1904, the neurotransmission phenomenon was postulated by Thomas Renton Elliot (1877–1961) and his mentor John Newport Langley (1852–1925).

Neurotransmitters are chemicals that allow transmission of signals from one neuron to the next across synapses. They are also found at the axon endings of neurons, where they stimulate the muscle fibres. Neurotransmitters must meet the following criteria to be classified as such:

• they must be present within a neuron;
• they must be released in response to neuron stimulation;
• they must have a post-synaptic receptor present.

Neurotransmitters can be excitatory or inhibitory. *Excitatory neurotransmitters* are the nervous system's 'on switches', increasing the likelihood of sending a signal that excites a neuron. They can be likened to the accelerator of a car – when pressed, it makes the car move or move faster. In other words, the excitatory transmitters act as the body's natural stimulants, generally serving to promote wakefulness, energy and activity. An example of an excitatory neurotransmitter is glutamate or adrenaline (see Table 4.2).

Neurotransmitter	Post-synaptic effect
Acetylcholine	Excitatory
GABA	Inhibitory
Glutamate	Excitatory
Dopamine	Excitatory/inhibitory
Serotonin	Excitatory/inhibitory
Adrenaline	Excitatory
Noradrenaline	Excitatory

Table 4.2: Classical neurotransmitters and their post-synaptic effects

Inhibitory neurotransmitters are the nervous system's 'off switches'. They decrease the likelihood of sending an excitatory signal. They can be likened to the brakes of a car – when pressed, they slow the car down or stop it moving. In other words, the inhibitory neurotransmitters act as the body's natural tranquillisers, generally serving to induce sleep, promote calmness and decrease aggression. The main inhibitory neurotransmitter is gamma-aminobutyric acid: GABA.

It has been proposed that there may be several hundred to several thousand neurotransmitters in the body, but only half a dozen or so are pharmacologically relevant and they are acetylcholine, serotonin, noradrenaline , adrenaline , dopamine, glutamate and GABA. These neurotransmitters are sometimes referred to as the classic neurotransmitters. In the long term, many more neurotransmitters may be discovered and many more will become pharmacologically important as new drugs are discovered.

Classic neurotransmitters

Neurotransmitters mediate neuron-to-neuron communication in the nervous system. Although these neurotransmitters show great diversity in many of their properties, they are all stored in small pockets called *vesicles* in nerve terminals and are released to the extracellular space or synapse. The action of neurotransmitters is terminated by reuptake or reabsorption back into presynaptic terminal or surrounding **glial cells** (see Figure 4.4). In certain instances the neurotransmitters are destroyed by enzymes instead of being reabsorbed back into the presynaptic neuron, a process called *catabolism*.

Acetylcholine

Acetylcholine was the first neurotransmitter to be identified. It is a neurotransmitter in both the peripheral and central nervous systems in many organisms, including humans. It is also the only neurotransmitter used in the motor division of the somatic nervous system. It activates muscles in the peripheral nervous system and is a major neurotransmitter in the autonomic nervous system. There are three acetylcholine pathways in the CNS:

* pons to thalamus and cortex;
* magnocellular forebrain nucleus to cortex;
* septohippocampal.

Adrenaline

Adrenaline, also known as epinephrine, is an excitatory neurotransmitter and hormone essential for the breakdown of fat. Adrenaline is derived from the compound noradrenaline (norepinephrine). As a neurotransmitter, adrenaline regulates attentiveness and mental focus. As a hormone, it is secreted along with noradrenaline, mainly in the medulla of the adrenal gland. Increased secretion of adrenaline can occur in response to fear or anger and will result in increased heart rate and the breakdown of glycogen to glucose. This reaction, commonly referred to as the 'fight or flight' response, prepares the body for strenuous activity. Adrenaline is used medicinally as a stimulant in cardiac arrest, as a vasoconstrictor in shock, as a bronchodilator and antispasmodic in bronchial asthma, and to counteract anaphylaxis. Commonly, adrenaline levels will be low due to adrenal fatigue (a pattern in which the adrenal output is suppressed due to chronic stress).

Therefore, symptoms can be presented as fatigue with low adrenaline levels. Low levels of adrenaline can also contribute to weight gain and poor concentration. Elevated levels of adrenaline can be factors contributing to restlessness, anxiety, sleep problems or acute stress.

Noradrenaline

Like adrenaline, noradrenaline is an excitatory neurotransmitter that is important for attention and focus. Noradrenaline is synthesised from *dopamine*. Levels of adrenaline in the CNS are only about 10 per cent of the levels of noradrenaline.

The noradrenergic system is most active when an individual is awake, which is important for focused attention. Increased noradrenaline activity seems to be a contributor to anxiousness. Also, brain noradrenaline turnover is increased in conditions of stress. Interestingly, *benzodiazepines*, which are the primary anxiolytic drugs, decrease firing of noradrenaline neurons. This may partly explain why benzodiazepines induce sleep.

Dopamine

Dopamine is an excitatory and inhibitory neurotransmitter, depending on the dopaminergic receptor it binds to. It is derived from the amino acid *tyrosine*. It is also the precursor to noradrenaline and adrenaline, which are all *catecholamines*, a group type of amino acids. Dopamine has many functions but plays a large role in the pleasure/reward pathway, affecting addiction thrills, memory and motor control. Like noradrenaline and adrenaline, it is stored in vesicles in the axon terminal. Dopamine plays a significant role in the cardiovascular, renal, hormonal and central nervous systems. The dopaminergic neurons have dendrites that extend into various regions of the brain, controlling different functions through the stimulation of adrenergic and dopaminergic receptors. Common symptoms with low dopamine levels are loss of motor control, addictions, cravings, compulsions and loss of satisfaction. When dopamine levels are elevated, symptoms may manifest in the form of anxiety, hyperactivity or psychosis.

Serotonin

Serotonin, or 5-hydroxytryptamine (5-HT), is a monoamine neurotransmitter that is primarily found in the gastrointestinal tract and CNS. Approximately 80 per cent of the human body's total serotonin is located in the gut, where it is used to regulate intestinal movements. The remainder is synthesised in serotonin neurons in the CNS. Serotonin is an excitatory and inhibitory neurotransmitter and acts as a target for symptoms such as low mood, compulsions, anxiousness and headaches, also affecting appetite, sleep, muscle contraction and some cognitive functions, including memory and learning.

Glutamate

Glutamate is the most abundant excitatory neurotransmitter in the human nervous system and it is necessary for memory and learning. It is believed that 70 per cent of the fast excitatory CNS synapses use glutamate as a transmitter. Excitatory neurotransmitters increase the activity of signal-receiving neurons and play a major role in controlling brain function. Glutamate exerts its effects on cells, in part, by binding to at least three neuroreceptors: the kainate, alpha-amino-

3-hydroxy-5-methyl-4-isoxazolepropionic acid (AMPA), and N-methyl-D-aspartate (NMDA) receptors, and activating these neuroreceptors results in excitation. Of these, the NMDA receptor plays a particularly important role in controlling the brain's ability to adapt to environmental and genetic influences, which is important for learning and memory.

An event or process that dramatically increases the activity of glutamate often increases the degree of neuronal excitation and, in extreme cases, can induce the death of neurons. Such a scenario is believed to take place in conditions such as ischemia, trauma, hypoxia, **hypoglycaemia**, and hepatic encephalopathy. Milder but chronic dysfunction of glutamate systems may play an important role in many neurodegenerative diseases, such as Huntington's chorea, disease or disorder (HD), Parkinson's, Alzheimer's, vascular dementia, and Tourette's and Korsakoff syndromes. Now turn to Activity 4.6 to test your understanding of what you have read in this section.

Activity 4.6

- Name the classical neurotransmitters that are excitatory and inhibitory.
- Can you explain the difference between the two types of neurotransmitters?

An outline answer is provided at the end of the chapter.

Gamma-aminobutyric acid

GABA is the major inhibitory neurotransmitter of the brain, occurring in 30–40 per cent of all synapses. The GABA concentration in the brain is 200–1,000 times greater than that of the adrenaline, noradrenaline, dopamine, serotonin or acetylcholine neurotransmitters.

It helps to induce relaxation and sleep, and balances the brain by inhibiting overexcitation of the neurons, contributing to motor control, vision and many other cortical functions. Anxiety is also regulated by GABA and some drugs that increase the level of GABA in the brain are used to treat epilepsy and to calm the trembling of people suffering from Huntington's chorea.

GABA also stimulates the anterior pituitary, leading to higher levels of human growth hormone (HGH), a hormone that contributes significantly to muscle growth and also prevents the creation of fat cells. To fully understand the role of neurotransmitters, we need to turn our attention to how a neurotransmitter impulse is generated.

Classic neurotransmission

Classic neurotransmission starts with a process called an *action potential* (see Figure 4.5). This is the difference in voltage between the inside and outside of a neuron membrane. In turn, the difference in voltage is caused by differences in electrically charges particles called *ions*. Examples of ions are sodium, potassium, chloride, calcium and magnesium ions. When a cell is in an unstimulated state, the concentration of sodium ions is greater outside the cell membrane than inside. Simultaneously, the concentration of potassium ions is greater inside the neuron than outside. In this unstimulated state, the neuron is said to be at its *resting potential* and its voltage is

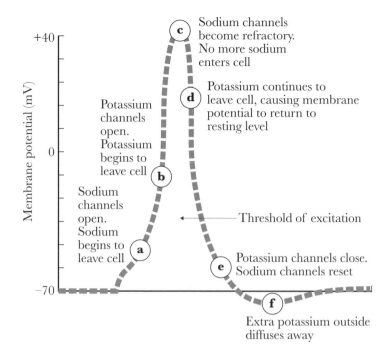

Figure 4.5: The generation of an action potential in a neuron

−70 millivolts (mV). At this resting potential the neuron is said to be *polarised* and its ion channels (pores that allows movement of ions in and out of the cell) are closed. This situation changes when a neuron is stimulated.

The stimulation of a neuron above a particular threshold will result in the opening of sodium channels, allowing sodium to rush inside the neuron causing a brief positive charge. At this point, the electrical *membrane potential* (see Figure 4.5) of the cell rapidly rises and falls, and this spike is called the action potential. The sodium channels then close; simultaneously, potassium channels open, allowing potassium ions to move out, therefore causing the membrane potential to go back to normal. The cell is now said to be *repolarised*. The potassium channels then close.

Before the membrane potential stabilises at −70mV there is a small undershoot called the *refractory period*. During this period, the neuron cannot fire another action potential. At this resting state (−70mV), the excess sodium and potassium ions will slowly diffuse away from the membrane and the neuron is ready to fire another action potential; once fired, the action potential quickly spreads along the axon like a wave until it reaches the axon terminal where chemical neurotransmission begins.

When an electrical impulse or action potential reaches the axon terminal, it is converted into a chemical messenger that is then released into the synapse. In the synapse, the neurotransmitters bind to receptors on the post-synaptic neuron, initiating an action potential in the adjacent neuron. An important point to remember here is that communication inside a neuron is electrical in nature, but communication between neurons is chemical in nature. Now that you have read this section, it is time to test your understanding by working on Activity 4.7.

Activity 4.7　　　　　　　*Evidence-based practice and research*

In a group or alone, research psychiatric illnesses that are a result of a shortage of one of the excitatory neurotransmitters. For each illness, list the neurotransmitter that is implicated.

An outline answer is provided at the end of the chapter.

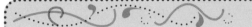

Chapter summary

Contrary to popular belief, the brain is not an organ. It is the most complex structure in our body and, although our knowledge of the brain has greatly increased thanks largely to new technology, there is a great deal we still do not know about this important structure. Currently, we know that the brain is divided into two hemispheres, which in turn are divided into the frontal, parietal, occipital and temporal lobes. In addition, the brain has two layers, namely the grey and white matter.

The basic cell of the brain is called the neuron and these are of many different shapes and sizes. They are mainly involved in cell-to-cell communication but, at times, the cells miscommunicate. The reason for this miscommunication is partly due to the wrong types of neurons making the wrong connections during a period of neural migration at prenatal development level. Neural miscommunication can result in neurodevelopmental conditions or psychiatric symptoms.

Neural communication is aided by chemicals at the synapse called neurotransmitters; there may be thousands of different types of these in the body, but only seven are currently of pharmacological importance: acetylcholine, GABA, glutamate, dopamine, serotonin, adrenaline and noradrenaline . Most medicines used to treat mental health problems work on these neurotransmitters.

Activities: brief outline answers

Activity 4.1 Clinical death (page 85)

If there is no electrical activity in the brainstem, it is possible to pronounce someone as clinically dead. The brainstem relays nerve impulses to the rest of the body. In particular, the medulla part of the brainstem is responsible for maintaining reflexes such as blood flow pressure, heart rate and breathing. If this is not happening, the individual is clinically dead.

Activity 4.2 Functions of the diencephalon (page 87)

The three main functions of the diencephalon are gating and processing sensory information; processing information involved in movement; and motivation and seeking reward.

Activity 4.3 The cerebral cortex (page 88)

The cerebral cortex is divided into hemispheres, which, in turn, are divided into lobes:

- frontal lobe: higher order functioning, critical thinking, memory including attention, planning, language and movement;
- parietal lobe: processing of sensory information;
- occipital lobe: vision;
- temporal lobes: sound and language.

Activity 4.4 Illnesses and brain dysfunction (page 90)

Illnesses associated with dysfunction of different areas of the brain are:

- cerebral cortex   depression, Huntington's chorea, mania;
- amygdala   depression;
- hippocampus   Alzheimer's disease, mania;
- pons   sleep disturbance;
- substantia nigra   Parkinson's disease.

Activity 4.5 Age of onset for psychosis (page 93)

Most psychosis, especially schizophrenia, starts in the late teens and early adulthood. This coincides with higher rates of neural pruning, whereby new connections are being made at various synapses in the brain.

Activity 4.6 Excitatory and inhibitory neurotransmitters (page 96)

- Excitatory: glutamate, dopamine, serotonin, adrenaline, noradrenaline, acetylcholine.
- Inhibitory: dopamine, GABA, serotonin.

Activity 4.7 Shortage of neurotransmitters (page 98)

- Dopamine   depression/psychosis
- Adrenaline   depression
- Serotonin   depression
- Glutamate   psychosis

Further reading

Gibb, B (2007) *The Rough Guide to the Brain*. New York: Rough Guides.

An accessible introduction to how the brain evolved and how it works.

Useful websites

www.neurogenesis.com/Neuroscience/index.php

This is a useful website that explains in very simple terms the concept of neural development.

www.neuroskills.com/brain.shtml

This is a useful website that explains in more detail about the different parts of the brain and their function. It has useful colour diagrams.

www.waiting.com/brainanatomy.html

Another useful website that explains the brain anatomy and very clearly anoted diagrams.

Chapter 5
Management and treatment of depression

NMC Standards for Pre-registration Nursing Education

This chapter will address the following competencies:

Domain 3: Nursing practice and decision-making

6.1 Mental health nurses must help people experiencing mental health problems to make informed choices about pharmacological and physical treatments, by providing education and information on the benefits and unwanted effects, choices and alternatives. They must support people to identify actions that promote health and help to balance benefits and unwanted effects.

7.1 Mental health nurses must provide support and therapeutic interventions for people experiencing critical and acute mental health problems. They must recognise the health and social factors that can contribute to crisis and relapse and use skills in early intervention, crisis resolution and relapse management in a way that ensures safety and security and promotes recovery.

8.1 Mental health nurses must practise in a way that promotes the self-determination and expertise of people with mental health problems, using a range of approaches and tools that aid wellness and recovery and enable self-care and self-management.

NMC Essential Skills Clusters

This chapter will address the following ESCs:

Cluster: Medicines management

36. People can trust the newly registered graduate nurse to ensure safe and effective practice in medicines management through comprehensive knowledge of medicines, their actions, risks and benefits.

40. People can trust a newly registered graduate nurse to work in partnership with people receiving medical treatments and their carers.

Chapter aims

By the end of this chapter, you should be able to:

- understand the main clinical features of depression;
- describe the neurotransmitters involved in depression;
- outline different classes of antidepressants and their action;
- understand antidepressant side effects and their management;
- choose the most appropriate antidepressant for a patient;
- know which common errors to avoid in the treatment of depression;
- understand what information to give the patient.

Introduction

Case study

George, a 52-year-old who was made redundant six months ago, has visited his GP complaining of intermittent headaches, fatigue and generalised lower back pain during the previous eight weeks. He has also reported that he has been sleeping a lot but that his sleep pattern is fractured. As a result, he does not feel refreshed after sleeping and he wakes up very early in the morning. He admits to having experienced stress some years back but does not acknowledge that he suffered from depression then. He does not feel sad but lately finds it increasingly difficult to cope with the behaviour of people around him. He denies abusing alcohol and reports that his drinking patterns and amounts of alcohol consumed have not changed. However, his wife reports that, for at least four months, her husband has been extremely irritable and difficult to rouse in the morning. She notices a definite increase in his alcohol consumption, estimating that he now has a few shots of whisky every night. The GP has suggested to George that he might be suffering from depression and has prescribed antidepressants, also referring George for counselling.

Depression as an illness has always existed and was recognised as far back as biblical times. According to the Old Testament, King Saul suffered from depression and committed suicide as a result. To better understand our current attitudes towards mental illness it is necessary to look back at prevailing attitudes during ancient times. At that time, it was believed that depression was caused by supernatural forces. Indeed, ancient human skulls have been found with large holes in them caused by drilling into the skull in an attempt to let evil spirits out. Thankfully, nowadays there is treatment for this illness, but before discussing the treatment of depression in detail, it is important for you to understand that not all forms of depression require antidepressants. It is important to distinguish different forms of depression and which particular forms will benefit the most from pharmacological strategies.

The mildest form of low mood is *reactive sadness*, which is when a person is emotionally reacting to some event that has happened in their lives; this can last for a few hours or a few days. Second in terms of severity is the concept of *grief*. This is a reaction to a major loss in a person's life and this response is normal. Situations that can cause grief range from divorce or separation from a loved one to bereavement. Grief usually last for months, but it is common for some people to experience grief for several years. The third type is *clinical depression*, which is a pathological condition characterised by loss of normal function in society, among other symptoms. It is this type of depression we are concerned with in this chapter.

This chapter will start with an overview of the hypothesis that underlines depression, before listing common physical disorders and medication that cause depression. Different classes of anti-depressants, their modes of action and side effects are covered in slightly more detail, followed by an overview of side-effects management. The final sections deal with common treatment errors that should be avoided and what the patient needs to know about the treatment. You will need to understand these theories as they form the bedrock of knowing how antidepressants work.

The monoamine hypothesis of depression

Before reading further, you need to refer to Chapter 4 and read about classical neurotransmitters and their functions.

Activity 5.1	*Critical thinking*

Are the neurotransmitters implicated in depression excitatory or inhibitory?

An outline answer is provided at the end of the chapter.

Scientific studies have found that numerous brain areas show altered activity in depressed patients. From a biological viewpoint, it has so far not been possible to determine a single area of the brain that causes depression. Research on the brains of depressed patients usually shows disturbed patterns of interaction between multiple parts of the brain. The areas that are most strongly affected are the raphe nuclei, suprachiasmatic nucleus, hypothalamic-pituitary-adrenal (HPA) axis, ventral tegmental area (VTA), nucleus accumbens (NAcc) and anterior cingulate cortex (ACC). It is hypothesised that depression is due to neurotransmitter malfunction in some or all of these parts of the brain.

There are at least three classical neurotransmitters implicated in depression: noradrenaline, serotonin and dopamine. Initially, there was some debate about which of these neurotransmitters is the most important in depression, but it is now generally accepted that all three are equally important. More recently, neuroprotective protein and the stress hormone cortisol have been shown to play a part in depression, although there is some debate about the mechanism.

The classical monoamine hypothesis of depression states that depression is due to low concentrations of these three monoamine neurotransmitters (noradrenaline, serotonin and dopamine) in the synapse. This theory was based on the observation that certain drugs, such as reserpine, that reduce the concentration of monoamine neurotransmitters in the brain can induce clinical depression. Mood elation, in contrast, may be associated with an excess of monoamine neuro-transmitters. Evidence supporting this hypothesis includes data from pharmacological studies, mainly in animals, suggesting that the actions of both major classes of antidepressant medicines work via the monoamines. As we will see later, the monoamine oxidase inhibitors (MAOIs) work by increasing brain concentrations of monoamines.

However, in recent times, the monoamine hypothesis has been challenged after the discovery that not all patients with depression have reduced monoamine levels in the synapse. Moreover, some people who are not depressed, but who exhibit violent or impulsive behaviour, have been found to have reduced levels of monoamines. This discovery has led to the modification of the classical hypothesis to one that includes neuroreceptors.

The monoamine receptor hypothesis

The monoamine receptor hypothesis of depression simply suggests that low concentrations of monoamine neurotransmitters lead to low activity levels at the synapse. In turn, this results in an increase in the number of post-synaptic receptors as a way of compensating for the reduced activity. This increase is called *receptor upregulation*. Upregulation coincides with the emergence of clinical symptoms of depression. Whatever the type of antidepressants, they all work by increasing the concentration of monoamine neurotransmitters in the synapse.

When an individual with depression responds to antidepressant treatment, the number of post-synaptic receptors decreases back to normal, a process called *receptor downregulation*. During upregulation, the patient develops a variety of symptoms and some patients may experience some or most of the following symptoms.

Symptoms of depression

The symptoms of depression can be many and varied, but these are the most commonly encountered:

- depressive mood
- apathy/loss of interest in daily activities
- decrease in normal functioning (work, social life)
- decreased self-esteem
- feelings of hopelessness
- feelings of guilt and worthlessness
- agitation and irritability
- suicidal ideation
- fatigue
- poor concentration
- poor appetite
- poor sleep pattern

For details of symptoms, please consult a textbook on psychopathology (several are listed at the end of the chapter).

Apart from social factors that trigger depression, there are some physical illnesses known to cause depression and it is those we will deal with next.

Common disorders known to cause depression

Some medical conditions, in certain situations, can trigger biochemical changes that can ultimately affect neurotransmission of the identified monoamines in a way that causes depression. Conditions such as influenza and thyroid disorder (**hypothyroidism**) are clear examples. For this reason, it is good practice to screen for thyroid function when a person presents with a mood disorder, as it is estimated that up to 10 per cent of all major depression is a result of low levels of thyroxine. The following list of common physical disorders associated with depression is not exhaustive, but provides you with an overview:

- vitamin deficiencies (B_{12}, niacin, thiamine)
- HIV/AIDS
- inflammatory disorders
- thyroid disorders
- cerebral vascular disease
- Addison's disease
- asthma
- chronic pain
- hepatitis
- diabetes

- **Cushing's syndrome**
- chronic fatigue syndrome
- syphilis
- influenza
- multiple sclerosis
- Parkinson's disease
- post-partum hormonal changes
- systemic lupus erythematosis
- porphyria

Drugs that may cause depression

Case study

Fred is a 27-year-old gym instructor who was referred to a psychiatrist by his GP because his depression had not shown any improvement despite his being on fluoxetine for 12 weeks. During his interview with the psychiatrist, Fred revealed for the first time that he was taking anabolic steroids to aid muscle building. The psychiatrist informed him that the anabolic steroids may have played a significant part in his depression and therefore advised against taking them. Fred stopped taking anabolic steroids and his mood gradually improved. He continued to take antidepressants for six months and he gradually weaned himself off them. He has not had a recurrence of depression ever since.

Some therapeutic and non-therapeutic medicines unfortunately may cause depression as a side effect. Recreational substances such as alcohol and drugs such as those in the case study above are known to alter mood and, therefore, it is important for you to routinely elicit information about the use of drugs or alcohol when you assess a patient. It is common for people with depression to use alcohol as a mood stimulant, but this is only a temporary measure as alcohol usually worsens mood. Also, it is common for people suffering from depression to increase their caffeine intake as a way of overcoming fatigue; caffeine also has some mild but transient antidepressant properties. This might sound like a good idea initially, but excess caffeine also causes sleeplessness, which in turn will retard recovery from depression. Some of the drugs and substances known to cause depression are:

- anti-hypertensives
- corticosteroids and other hormones
- anti-Parkinson's drugs (levodopa, carbidopa)
- anxiolytic drugs (diazepam, etc.)
- birth control pills
- alcohol

- sedatives
- barbiturates
- appetite suppressants
- analgesics
- antibacterial and antifungal drugs
- antineoplastic drugs

Classes of antidepressants and their side effects

In many respects, the discovery of antidepressants could be regarded as accidental. Researchers carrying out trials on new medication to treat tuberculosis in the 1950s found that the medication had mood-elevating effects. This initial discovery led to the creation of two classes of first-generation antidepressants: tricyclic antidepressants (TCAs) and MAOIs. More recently, the selective serotonin reuptake inhibitors (SSRIs) form the second and third generations of antidepressants, collectively known as serotonin-noradrenaline reuptake inhibitors (SNRIs), and were introduced during the 1990s.

Tricyclic antidepressants

TCAs have an important place in the treatment history of depression as they were the first such medicines to be discovered. It is their mode of action that helped to formulate theories of depression and, for many years, TCAs were the first-line treatment of clinical depression. Although they are still considered to be highly effective, they have been increasingly replaced by the SSRIs and other newer antidepressants. Nonetheless, TCAs are still occasionally used for treatment-resistant depression that has failed to respond to therapy with newer antidepressants. TCAs are also indicated for treatment of secondary depression in other illnesses such as psychosis and dementia, depression with anxiety and post-stroke depression. They are not considered addictive and are somewhat preferable to the MAOIs. Patients usually experience the side effects of the TCAs before the therapeutic benefits, and for this reason they may potentially be dangerous, as willpower can be increased, possibly giving the patient a greater energy and power to attempt or commit suicide. In this regard the dosages of TCAs should be carefully monitored.

Mode of action of TCAs

TCAs work by preventing the absorption of monoamine neurotransmitters in the synapse back into the the presynaptic neuron (see Figure 4.4 on page 92). Most TCAs tend to act mainly as SNRIs by inhibiting the serotonin transporter (SERT) and the noradrenaline transporter (NAT), respectively. The disabling of these two transport systems results in the accumulation of serotonin and noradrenaline in the synapse, therefore enhancing the chances of neurotransmission. Although the monoamine dopamine has been implicated in depression, TCAs have very little

Generic name	Noradrenaline	Serotonin	Monoamine oxidase	Dopamine
Imipramine	++	+++	–	0
Desipramine	++++	0	0	0
Amitryptiline	+	++++	0	0
Nortriptyline	+++	++	0	0
Trimipramine	++	++	0	0
Doxepin	+++	++	0	0
Clomipramine	+++	+++++	–	–

Table 5.1: Tricyclic antidepressants, showing types of neurotransmitters they act on (the more plus signs, the greater the action)

action on the dopamine transporter (DAT), and therefore have very little efficacy as dopamine reuptake inhibitors (DRIs) (see Table 5.1).

The best way to start TCAs is by employing a low dose and increasing every three to five days. Most TCAs have a linear pharmcokinetics profile; in other words, a change in dose will lead to a proportional change in the blood serum level. Once the blood serum level reaches **steady state**, the dosage of a TCA can be given as a single dose before bedtime because they have a relatively long half-life. They show therapeutic effects within 7–28 days and, at times, patients may lose response to antidepressants after several months, a condition called *poop-out syndrome*.

Side effects of TCAs

Apart from their role in inhibiting neurotransmitter transport systems, many TCAs also have a high affinity as antagonists at specific receptor sites, such as the various serotonin and alpha$_1$-adrenergic receptors, some of which may contribute to their therapeutic efficacy, as well as their side effects. For example, they have varying but typically high affinity for antagonising the H$_1$ and H$_2$ histamine receptors, resulting in weight gain and drowsiness. They also antagonise the muscarinic acetylcholine receptors and this leads to adverse side effects such as constipation, dry mouth, blurred vision, dry nose, urinary retention and cognitive impairment. Most, if not all, TCAs are potent inhibitors of sodium channels, which accounts for their adverse cardiac effects, but can also explain their beneficial effects on neuropathic pain.

Other common side effects of TCAs include anxiety, emotional blunting (apathy/**anhedonia**), confusion, restlessness, akathisia, hypersensitivity, sweating, sexual dysfunction, muscle twitches, weakness, nausea and vomiting, tachycardia and, rarely, irregular heart rhythms. A condition called rhabdomyolysis, or muscle breakdown, has been reported in very rare cases with this class of antidepressants. Tolerance to these adverse effects often develops if treatment is continued. Side effects may also be less troublesome if treatment is initiated with low doses and then gradually increased, although this may also delay the beneficial effects.

One of the most important side effects of TCAs is a reduction in the heart rhythm (arrythmia), so they can, in theory, stop contraction of heart muscle fibres, decrease cardiac contractility and increase collateral blood circulation to ischemic heart muscle. Naturally, in overdose, they are cardiotoxic, prolonging heart rhythms and increasing myocardial irritability. Antidepressants in general may produce a *discontinuation syndrome*. This is not the same as drug withdrawal and this will be explained in later sections.

Monoamine oxidase inhibitors

MAOIs were the second type of antidepressants developed after TCAs. Their use is restricted because of their unfavourable safety profile; they have mostly been replaced by the newer and safer SSRIs and other safe non-SSRIs or atypical antidepressants.

Mode of action of MAOIs

The monoamine neurotransmitters, namely serotonin, noradrenaline and dopamine, are released into the synaptic cleft, where they transmit chemical messages by binding to the post-synaptic receptors (see Figure 4.4 on page 92). After transmitting messages, some of monoamines are reabsorbed back into the presynaptic neuron or they are destroyed. The destruction of these neurotransmitters is catalysed by an enzyme called *monoamine oxidase* (MAO). MAOIs work by stopping this enzyme from catalysing the destruction of neurotransmitters, resulting in the accumulation of monoamines in the synaptic cleft.

The enzyme MAO has another role in the brain – it controls levels of *tyramine*, a chemical that is associated with causing high blood pressure and headaches. When an MAOI medicine inhibits MAO enzyme activity, it causes higher levels of tyramine, which in turn causes high blood pressure. A high spike in tyramine can lead to a sudden jump in blood pressure, called a *hypertensive crisis*, which can lead to stroke or even death.

The most significant risk associated with the use of MAOIs is the potential for interactions with over-the-counter and prescription medicines, illicit drugs or medications, and some herbal medicines, for example St John's wort (*Hypericum perforatum*). For this reason, many users carry an MAOI-card, which lets emergency medical personnel know what medicines to avoid. For example, if you are administering adrenaline to someone on MAOIs, you should reduce the dose by at least 75 per cent, and you should extend the duration for administration. Also, you should be aware that MAOI medications interact with other medicines or certain foods, and this can be particularly dangerous; this will be dealt with in other sections. Examples of foods and drinks with potentially high levels of tyramine include fermented substances, such as Chianti and other aged wines, and aged cheeses. Liver is also a well-known source of tyramine and some meat extracts and yeast extracts, such as Bovril, Marmite and Vegemite, contain extremely high levels of tyramine, and should not be used with these medications. Before you read the next section on the safety profile of these medicines, please try Activity 5.2.

Activity 5.2   *Evidence-based practice and research*

Consult a textbook or research on the internet the different type of foods that a patient should avoid eating while on MAOI therapy.

An outline answer is provided at the end of the chapter.

MAOIs should not be combined with other psychoactive substances, antidepressants, painkillers or stimulants, either legal or illegal. Certain combinations can cause lethal reactions, common examples including SSRIs, tricyclics, meperidine, tramadol and dextromethorphan.

Common side effects of MAOIs

As mentioned earlier, MAOIs interact with foods that contain tyramine and eating these foods can cause a hypertensive crisis. You should take emergency action if a patient on MAOIs reports or exhibits any of the following symptoms: severe chest pain, severe headache, stiff or sore neck, enlarged pupils, fast or slow heartbeat, increased sensitivity to light, increased sweating (possibly with fever or cold, clammy skin), nausea and vomiting.

Other common side effects of MAOI are blurred vision, urinary retention, sexual dysfunction, mild dizziness or light-headedness, especially when getting up from a lying or sitting position, drowsiness, mild headache, increased appetite followed by weight gain, increased sweating, muscle twitching during sleep, restlessness, shakiness or trembling, tiredness and weakness or trouble sleeping. Other side effects that are less common with MAOIs are chills, constipation, decreased appetite and dryness of mouth.

Selective serotonin reuptake inhibitors

SSRIs are a newer class of antidepressants. They are now widely used because of their favourable safety profile and they are at least as effective as the older TCAs. Like TCAs, SSRIs exert their function by increasing the concentration of monoamines in the synaptic cleft by inhibiting their reuptake (see Figure 4.4 on page 92). However, there is one notable difference: SSRIs selectively inhibit synaptic serotonin being pumped back into the presynaptic neuron, resulting in the accumulation of serotonin in the synaptic cleft. SSRIs have varying degrees of selectivity for the other monoamine transporters, with pure SSRIs having only weak affinity for the noradrenaline and dopamine transporters (see Table 5.2).

SSRIs have secondary pharmacological action other than the blocking of the serotonin reuptake pump. Indeed, no two SSRIs have identical secondary pharmacological actions, which might include noradrenaline reuptake blockade, dopamine reuptake blockade, serotonin $5HT_{2c}$ antagonism, muscarinic cholinergic antagonism and sigma$_1$ receptor actions. It is plausible that the secondary binding profile of SSRIs can account for differences in efficacy and tolerability in different patients. Serotonin actions at serotonin $5HT_{2c}$ receptors inhibit the release of both dopamine and noradrenaline; however, we know that medicines that block $5HT_{2c}$ receptors, such as fluoxetine, have the opposite effect, disinhibiting the release of dopamine and noradrenaline into the synapse. This may explain why many patients, even from the first dose, detect an energising and fatigue-reducing effect of fluoxetine that is accompanied by an improvement in concentration and attention. Some possible daily dosages of SSRIs are shown in Table 5.3.

Common side effects of SSRIs

In this section, we will deal with general side effects of SSRIs and it is important to note that most side effects are present during the first four weeks of treatment, at a time when the body is

Generic name	Noradrenaline	Serotonin	Monoamine oxidase	Dopamine
Fluoxetine	0	+ + + + +	0	0
Paroxetine	+	+ + + + +	0	0
Sertraline	0	+ + + + +	0	+
Fluvoxamine	0	+ + + + +	0	0
Citalopram	0	+ + + + +	0	0
Escitalopram	0	+ + + + +	0	0

Table 5.2: SSRIs, showing types of neurotramitters they act on (the more plus signs, the greater the action)

Generic name	Recommended daily dose
Citalopram	10–60mg
Escitolapram	5–20mg
Fluoxetine	20–80mg
Paroxetine	20–50mg
Fluvoxamine	50–300mg
Setraline	50–200mg

Table 5.3: A selection of SSRIs and possible daily dosages

adapting to the new medicine. The only exception to this is the occurrence of sexual side effects later in the course of treatment; in most cases, these occur between six to eight weeks after the medicine has been started. It is also during this period that the medicine begins to reach its full potential in terms of efficacy. In general, most SSRIs can cause one or more of the following symptoms: anhedonia, apathy, nausea and vomiting, drowsiness or headache, extremely vivid or strange dreams, dizziness, fatigue, pupil dilation (mydriasis), urinary retention, weight loss/gain, increased risk of bone fractures and injuries, increased feelings of depression and anxiety (which may sometimes provoke panic attacks), tremors (and other symptoms of Parkinsonism in vulnerable elderly patients), autonomic dysfunction, including **orthostatic hypotension**, increased or reduced sweating, akathisia, renal impairment, suicidal ideation (thoughts of suicide), photosensitivity and changes in sexual behaviour.

Sexual side effects

SSRIs can cause various forms of sexual dysfunction, such as inability to achieve an orgasm, erectile dysfunction and diminished sexual appetite. Recent evidence suggests that such side effects occur in 17–41 per cent of patients (Landen et al., 2005). Side effects of these antidepressants are brought about by the stimulation of postsynaptic $5\text{-}HT_2$ and $5\text{-}HT_3$ receptors. The stimulation of these serotonin receptor subtypes leads to a decrease in dopamine and noradrenaline release from the substantia nigra, leading to sexual dysfunction.

SSRI discontinuation syndrome

> ### Case study
>
> *Megan is 43 years old and suffers from depression. She has been taking paroxetine 60mg a day for eight weeks. Because she feels a lot better, she asked her doctor to be on a lower dose and the doctor tapered off the dose in 20mg decrements. Within a couple of days of dose reduction, she started to show severe flu-like symptoms – headache, diarrhoea, nausea, vomiting, chills, dizziness, fatigue and insomnia, agitation, impaired concentration, vivid dreams, depersonalisation, irritability and suicidal thoughts.*

SSRI discontinuation syndrome is a condition that can occur following dosage reduction, discontinuation or interruption of mainly SSRIs or SNRI antidepressants. The condition typically starts from the time of reduction in dosage or complete discontinuation, depending on the half-life of the medicine and the patient's metabolism. Currently, there is no universally acceptable definition of SSRI discontinuation syndrome, but Schatzberg et al. (1997) have noted that:

> *SSRI discontinuation symptoms . . . may emerge when an SSRI is abruptly discontinued, when doses are missed, and less frequently, during dosage reduction. In addition, the symptoms are not attributable to any other cause and can be reversed when the original agent is reinstituted, or one that is pharmacologically similar is substituted . . . Physical symptoms include problems with balance, gastrointestinal and flu-like symptoms, and sensory and sleep disturbances. Psychological symptoms include anxiety and/or agitation, crying spells, irritability and aggressiveness.*

Symptoms of the syndrome are many and varied and, apart from those mentioned above, can include dizziness, electric shock-like sensations, sweating, nausea, insomnia, tremor, confusion, nightmares and vertigo. The precise mechanism of SSRI discontinuation syndrome is yet to be discovered but suggestions include electrophysiological changes in the brain and body, as well as dopamine dependency or an overexcited immune system.

SSRIs with a short half-life are more likely to cause discontinuation syndrome. Those SSRIs with a long half-life, such as fluoxetine, are associated less with the syndrome. Because of its long half-life, fluoxetine has been used in the treatment of discontinuation syndrome and this can be done either by administering a single 20mg dose or by starting the patient on a low dose and slowly **titrating** down.

Suicidality in children and adolescents

There is increasing evidence that SSRIs can increase the risk of suicidality in children and adolescents (Olfson et al., 2006). In 2004, the US Food and Drug Administration (FDA) pooled studies and found a statistically significant increase of up to 80 per cent risk of *possible suicidal ideation and suicidal behaviour* and an increase of up to 130 per cent of agitation in children and adolescents. Also in 2004, the UK Medicines and Healthcare products Regulatory Agency (MHRA) judged fluoxetine (Prozac) to be the only antidepressant that offered a favourable risk–benefit ratio in children with depression, although it was also associated with a slight increase in the risk of self-harm and suicidal ideation. In the UK, only sertraline and fluvoxamine are licensed for use with children and only for the treatment of obsessive-compulsive disorder (OCD). Fluoxetine, despite having a favourable risk–benefit ratio for use with depression in adolescents and children, is not licensed for this use.

Atypical antidepressants

In addition to the antidepressants described so far, there is a range of antidepressants that work in increasingly more complex ways, including serotonin-noradrenaline reuptake inhibitors (SNRIs), noradrenaline reuptake inhibitors (NRIs), noradrenaline dopamine reuptake inhibitors (NDRIs) and serotonin antagonist reuptake inhibitors (SARIs). Of these classes, we will cover the SNRIs in more detail because of their increasing popularity.

Serotonin–noradrenaline reuptake inhibitors

SNRIs work by inhibiting the reuptake of the neurotransmitters serotonin and noradrenaline. This results in an increase in concentration of serotonin and noradrenaline in the synaptic cleft and therefore an increase in neurotransmission. Most SNRIs, including venlafaxine, desvenlafaxine and duloxetine, are several times more selective for serotonin over noradrenaline, while milnacipran is three times more selective for noradrenaline than serotonin. A property of SNRIs that they share with older TCAs is that they are effective against neuropathic pain.

The SNRIs were developed more recently than the SSRIs and, as a result, there are relatively few of them. However, the SNRIs are among the most widely used antidepressants today because they have demonstrated slightly higher antidepressant efficacy than the SSRIs (apparently owing to their dual mechanism) and because their side effects are slightly less severe.

Because the SNRIs and SSRIs both act similarly to elevate serotonin levels, they subsequently share many of the side effects, although to varying degrees. The most common include loss of appetite, weight and sleep. There may also be drowsiness, dizziness, fatigue, headache, mydriasis, nausea and vomiting, sexual dysfunction and urinary retention. There are two common sexual side effects: diminished interest in sex (libido) and difficulty reaching climax (anorgasmia), which are usually somewhat milder with the SNRIs in comparison to the SSRIs. Nonetheless, sexual side effects account for lack of adherence to both SSRIs and SNRIs.

Treatment and management of depression

A range of psychological and psychosocial interventions for depression have been shown to relieve the symptoms of the condition and there is growing evidence that psychosocial therapies can help people recover from depression in the longer term (NICE, 2009b). However, not everyone responds adequately to psychosocial therapies and, for those who do not, the use of antidepressants may be a viable alternative as their effectiveness has long been recognised.

The severity of depression for which antidepressants show consistent benefits is at present poorly defined but, in general, the more severe the symptoms, the greater the benefit (Anderson et al., 2008). Antidepressants are normally recommended as first-line treatment in patients whose depression is of at least moderate to severe and, out of this group, approximately 20 per cent will respond with no treatment at all, 30 per cent will respond to a placebo and 50 per cent will respond to antidepressant drugs (NICE, 2009b).

Until recently, we have believed that antidepressants take about two to four weeks to begin to work. This has recently been challenged, as evidence from clinical trials shows that symptom improvement can start immediately, with the greatest degree of improvement occurring in the first week. Posternak and Zimmerman (2005) conducted a meta-analysis of 47 studies and found that 35 per cent of the improvement occurred between weeks 0 and 1, and 25 per cent between weeks 1 and 2. It is still important to emphasise to your patient that antidepressants in general can take a long time to take effect. What we now know is that antidepressant effects can be immediate in some people, or it can take up to eight weeks or more in others. A large study called Sequenced Treatment Alternatives to Relieve Depression (STAR*D) enrolled 2,876 patients, followed up to 12 weeks, and found that the average response time to antidepressants was 5.7 weeks. However, in some cases, the average response time for patients on antidepressants can be longer, as evidenced by a large and influential naturalistic study (Trivedi et al., 2006).

Choice of antidepressant

No antidepressant has been consistently proved to be superior to another, but they do differ in their side effects profiles and this can usually be the determining factor in choosing an anti-depressant. In this regard, you need to discuss antidepressant treatment options with the patient, which should cover the choice of antidepressant and any possible side effects, for example insomnia, sexual side effects, discontinuation symptoms or sedation.

If the patient has been on antidepressants before, find out from them whether they were effective or not. The NICE guideline (2009b) recommends that the first-line antidepressant treatment should be an SSRI. This recommendation is made partly due to these medicines' reduced risk profile and because they are just as effective as other antidepressants. However, SSRIs are associated with an increased risk of bleeding, especially in older people or those taking other medicines that have the potential to damage the gastrointestinal mucosa or interfere with clotting. These include herbal medicines such as *Ginkgo biloba*.

In certain cases, patients may not show improvement with one class of antidepressant and, in such cases, it may be preferable to switch to a different type.

Activity 5.3   *Critical thinking*

Bill is a 57-year-old man who presented to his GP with depression, complaining of low mood, loss of energy and concentration, and poor appetite. He was prescribed amitryptline 50mg to be taken twice a day. After six weeks, Bill has approached a nurse to say that his depression has hardly changed and, if anything, he feels worse. Bill is worried about the sedation and the lack of energy he has been experiencing. He asks you for your view regarding medication. What would you advise Bill to do?

An outline answer is provided at the end of the chapter.

Antidepressants are generally prescribed using lower doses to start with and then gradually increasing the dose. Adults between the ages of 16 and 55 years should receive doses within the recommended range, with adults over the age of 55 receiving lower doses.

The treatment of depression can be roughly divided into three phases: acute, continuation and maintenance treatment. Acute treatment will usually begin with the first dose and extends until the patient no longer has symptoms, and this may take up to eight weeks. The next phase will be the continuation phase during which treatment is maintained to avoid relapse of symptoms, and this can last up to six months beyond the acute phase. You should advise your patient to remain on the same dose for maximum effect. Available evidence suggests that a patient should be maintained on the same dose that was used during the acute stages of the illness for maximum effect.

In first-episode depression the dose can gradually be reduced at the end of the acute phase. You should inform your patient that gradual withdrawal of antidepressants is very important in order to prevent discontinuation syndrome, a condition that is caused by a sudden withdrawal of antidepressant treatment (see page 110 earlier in this chapter). After antidepressants have been withdrawn, you should advise the patient to be alert for any signs of relapse, such as poor sleep, tiredness or poor appetite. In the event of these symptoms recurring, you should advise the patient to contact a member of the healthcare team.

Available evidence suggests that those people whose depression occurred before the age of 18 years and who have a family history of mood disorders are likely to have a recurrence of the illness. In such cases, you should alert the patient that lifelong medication treatment may be recommended to avoid relapse. If these risk factors are absent, however, antidepressant treatment can gradually be discontinued. If a patient suffers three or more depressive episodes, lifelong medication treatment is recommended (NICE, 2009b).

Management of side effects

You will note that, in people who are suffering from depression, their feelings of hopelessness and pessimism are pervasive. But when depressed patients encounter troubling side effects, they are likely to discontinue taking medication, particularly where these side effects occur long before the patient enjoys the positive therapeutic effect of the medication. It is therefore important for you to know how to manage the common side effects and this is outlined below.

- **Postural hypotension**: This is low blood pressure that causes dizziness, especially on standing up quickly, and is more common in older patients and those with diabetes. Advise the patient not to stand up too quickly and also to drink lots of fluids. In some cases, special nylon stockings can be given to promote arterial constriction in the legs. In severe cases, medication such as noradrenaline and phenylephrine 9-a-fluorohydrocortisone can be given by mouth.
- **Sexual dysfunction**: This includes difficulties during any stage of normal sexual activity, including desire, arousal or orgasm. Encourage the patient to ask the doctor to switch to other antidepressant medication such as bupropion or nefazodone. In some cases, sildenafil citrate (Viagra) is effective for erectile dysfunction.
- **Drowsiness**: This includes sleepiness, fatigue, lethargy, exhaustion or sluggishness, lasting a few hours after taking the medication, most commonly TCAs. Advise the patient not to

drive or use machinery. If the patient is taking divided doses, taking a single large dose at night is preferable. Discuss the possibility of switching to antidepressants such as SSRIs or newer SNRIs. Advise the patient to drink plenty of fluids.

- **Constipation**: This involves bowel movements that are infrequent or hard to pass and is a common cause of painful defaecation, with a feeling of being 'bunged up'. Advise the patient to eat more foods with fibre such as fruit, green vegetables or bran. Prune or aloe vera juice can be useful. Advise plenty of fluids, regular meals and regular exercise, especially walking. If this does not help, the patient may have to ask the doctor to prescribe a laxative on a short-term basis.
- **Blurred vision**: The patient has difficulties in focusing with things looking fuzzy. Advise the patient not to drive. In some cases, pilocarpine eye drops can be prescribed. Reassure the patient that the effect is transient.
- **Xerostomia**: This is dry mouth, with not much saliva. The patient should avoid decongestants and antihistamines as they worsen the problem. Advise the patient to pay careful attention to oral hygiene and drink non-carbonated, sugarless fluids frequently; chewing xylitol-containing gum and using a carboxymethyl cellulose saliva substitute as a mouthwash may help. Pilocarpine may be prescribed and oxidised glycerol triesters treatment is sometimes used to coat the mouth.
- **Weight gain**: An increase in body weight may be due to either an increase in muscle mass, fat deposits or excess fluids such as water. Encourage a well-balanced diet rich in vegetables, fibre and fruit, and regular cardiovascular exercise, such as walking or swimming. Advise the patient to ask the doctor to prescribe other antidepressants instead, such as some SSRIs or bupropion.
- **Tremors**: These are involuntary, rhythmic muscle contractions and relaxation involving to-and-fro movements of one or more body parts, most common with SSRIs. Arrange for the patient to be seen by a doctor.
- **Skin rashes**: The skin changes its colour, appearance or texture and this may be localised or all over the body. The skin may itch, swell, or become warm, bumpy, dry, cracked or blistered, and it may be painful. Advise the patient to stop the medication and see a doctor as soon as possible.
- **Palpitations**: These are an abnormality of heartbeat that cause a conscious awareness of its beating. Reassure the patient that this is not dangerous and, if it persists, refer them to a doctor.
- **Urinary retention**: This is an inability to urinate, characterised by poor urinary stream with intermittent flow, straining or a sense of incomplete voiding and hesitancy. Arrange for the patient to see a doctor to review the medication. Bethanechol is sometimes given to relieve the symptoms.
- **Headache**: Advise the patient to drink lots of water; good ventilation is also helpful. Ask the patient to try paracetamol, and check for interaction with any other medication the patient might be taking.
- **Insomnia**: This is an inability to sleep during the night. Arrange for the patient to see the doctor to review medication. SSRIs are best taken in the morning and TCAs at night. Encourage exercise during the day, and advise against drinks and foods rich in caffeine. Advise the patient to drink hot chocolate or herbal drinks such as valerian tea before bedtime, and to sleep in a well-ventilated room.

- **Diarrhoea**: This is three or more loose, liquid bowel movements per day, more common with SSRIs. Advise the patient to drink plenty of water and, if it lasts more than a day, arrange for them to be seen by a doctor.
- **Restlessness or anxiety**: This is more common with SSRIs. Advise the patient to relax by taking deep breaths and exhaling slowly. The wearing of loose clothing might be helpful. A low starting dose of antidepressants can also be beneficial.

Overdose

SSRIs appear to be safer in overdose when compared with traditional antidepressants such as the TCAs. This relative safety is supported by both case series and studies of deaths per numbers of prescriptions. However, case reports of SSRI poisoning have indicated that severe toxicity can occur and deaths have been reported following massive single ingestions, although this is very uncommon when compared to the TCAs. Because of the wide therapeutic index of the SSRIs, most patients will have mild or no symptoms following moderate overdoses. The most commonly reported severe effect following SSRI overdose is *serotonin syndrome*.

Serotonin syndrome is a potentially life-threatening adverse reaction that may occur following therapeutic use of antidepressants. It is not an idiosyncratic medicine reaction, but predictable if there is an excess of serotonin in the CNS. Numerous medicines and medicine combinations have been reported to produce serotonin syndrome. The excess serotonin activity produces a spectrum of specific symptoms that include cognitive, autonomic and somatic effects and, in many cases, it produces symptoms that are not unlike those of neuroleptic malignant syndrome (see Chapter 7 on antipsychotics). The symptoms may range from barely perceptible to fatal. Other reported significant effects include coma, seizures and cardiac toxicity.

Treatment for SSRI overdose is mainly based on symptomatic and supportive care. Medical care may be required for agitation, maintenance of the airways, and treatment for serotonin syndrome. ECG monitoring is usually indicated to detect any cardiac abnormalities.

Common treatment errors to avoid

For patients who are depressed, restless and agitated, giving them SSRIs might worsen the symptoms. By contrast, TCAs may be indicated because of their sedative properties. Most SSRIs should be given in the morning to reduce the risk of insomnia. By contrast, TCAs can be given at night as a single dose to aid sleeping and to avoid daytime drowsiness. Many patients with depression are prone to non-adherence to medication and therefore strategies to improve adherence should be instituted with those at risk. You need to be particularly vigilant in those patients using illicit substances as the use of such substances, particularly alcohol, is a common reason why antidepressants lose their efficacy. Antidepressants should be allowed sufficient time to work and a patient can be on the same dose for up to eight weeks before review. Abrupt or rapid withdrawal of antidepressants should be avoided as this could result in the patient suffering from discontinuation syndrome. TCAs should be avoided in the elderly or those with a history of heart problems as they are cardiotoxic. The elderly are particularly vulnerable to developing heart conditions due to their use.

What the patient needs to know

- Tell the patient that, although psychological symptoms of depression may take up to four weeks to begin to improve, physical symptoms may start improving soon after commencement of treatment.
- Highlight to the patient subtle indicators of improvement if they are present during the early stages, such as being more relaxed, sleeping better, and appetite improvement. This should help the patient to feel positive.
- Tell the patient that they may experience side effects, and that these can best be managed by dose adjustment or by switching to another antidepressant.
- Advise the patient not drink alcohol while on antidepressants as alcohol can inhibit their effects.
- Advise the patient that antidepressants are not addictive but should not be withdrawn abruptly as this almost always leads to discontinuation syndrome.
- Advise the patient to take up exercise and refrain from taking stimulants such as alcohol or caffeine. These substances will impair sleep and this leads to prolonged or poor recovery from depression.
- Patients on MAOIs should be given a list of foods rich in tyramine that they should avoid.

Chapter summary

The main symptoms of depression are loss of appetite, poor sleep and concentration, low mood, lack of energy and suicidal feelings, among others. Most types of depression subside without pharmacological treatment but, in many cases, antidepressants are required.

Most antidepressants work by increasing levels of monoamine neurotransmitters in the synapse. The TCAs achieve this by stopping the absorption of these neurotransmitters back in the presynaptic neurone. The MAOIs achieve the same by inhibiting the enzyme that destroys these neurotransmitters, thereby increasing their concentration in the synapse. SSRIs are the first-line treatment because of their good safety profile, but other antidepressants can be used. All antidepressants are equally effective but differ in their side-effect profiles. Therefore, the choice of antidepressants should take into account safety and side effects. Antidepressants should never be stopped abruptly or discontinued too quickly for fear of discontinuation syndrome. MAOIs are restricted in their use because of their high-risk profile and because foods rich in tyramine should be avoided.

Activities: brief outline answers

Activity 5.1 Neurotransmitters (page 102)

In the case of depression, they are excitatory, therefore causing symptoms of depression.

Activity 5.2 Foods to avoid with MAOIs (page 107)

Banana peels, bean curd, broad (fava) bean pods, cheese, fish, ginseng, protein extracts, meat (non-fresh and liver), sausage, bologna, pepperoni, salami, sauerkraut, shrimp paste, soups and yeast.

Activity 5.3 Lack of energy and amitryptiline (page 112)

It very likely that Bill's lack of energy may have been exacerbated by the current medicine he is taking, amitryptiline. One of the side effects of this medicine is sedation, particularly if it is taken during the day, as in Bill's case. One option is for Bill to take a single dose of 100mg at night time or you should inform Bill of an SSRI or SNRI as an alternative option. These medicines are unlikely to cause sedation but you should warn Bill of the possibility of poor sleep, sexual dysfunction, or serotonin syndrome.

Further reading

Preston, JD, O'Neal, JH and Talaga, MC (2008) *A Handbook of Clinical Psychopharmacology*, 5th edition. Oakland, CA: New Harbinger Publications.

A clearly written book and particularly useful for those from a non-medical background. It explains non-pharmacological mental healthcare well.

Stahl, SM (2009) *Stahl's Essential Psychopharmacology: The prescriber's guide*, 3rd edition. Cambridge: Cambridge University Press.

A comprehensive guide to psychopharmacology that is clearly written and has good illustrations.

Taylor, D, Paton, C and Kapur, S (2009) *The Maudsley Prescribing Guidelines*, 10th edition. London: Informa Healthcare.

A very useful, easy-to-understand, evidence-based prescribing and general medicines management manual. It is particularly useful for prescribers.

Useful websites

www.depressionalliance.org

This website provides information and support to depression suffers.

www.mind.org.uk/help/diagnoses_and_conditions/depression

Again, this website provides information and support to sufferers and carers of people with depression.

www.nhs.uk/Conditions/Depression

An NHS website that provides information to patients, carers and professionals.

Chapter 6
Management and treatment of bipolar disorder

Introduction

Case study

Elizabeth is a 29-year-old married mother of two young children who presented with a history of recurrent and disabling depression. A few weeks before presentation, she became severely depressed and had difficulty moving because of loss of energy and appetite. She felt suicidal. At the time of presentation, she was prescribed the antidepressant paroxetine 30mg a day. In the past, she confessed to her mood lifting very quickly to the point of elation after being on a course of antidepressants for a relatively short time. For this reason, she found it unnecessary to continue taking her paroxetine but relapsed very quickly; hence, she was admitted to hospital. On admission to the ward, she was seen by a doctor who was keen to take a more detailed medical history of her and her family. She revealed that she fell off a horse and sustained concussion when she was 19 years old. She described a history of mood swings since the age of 13 and during her teens she had abused alcohol and recreational drugs. She also revealed that both her father and paternal grandmother suffered from mood swings. In particular, her paternal grandmother was hospitalised for an unspecified illness that the family refuses to talk about.

The doctor was unsure about the diagnosis of major depressive disorder given the pattern of her response to antidepressants. She was prescribed fluoxetine but this was discontinued because it appeared to worsen her underlying mood swings. The doctor suspected that Elizabeth was suffering from bipolar disorder and placed her on lithium carbonate 800mg a day. Within a week, she began to improve markedly, with clearer thinking, more productive work, less depression, fewer mood swings and more energy. Within five weeks of treatment with lithium carbonate Elizabeth felt 'terrific'. She was referred for supportive psychotherapy, which helped her to settle down and gave her more confidence and a feeling of control over her life.

Mood disorders have been recognised as early as the fifth century BC. Hippocrates was the first physician to recognise that mood disorders are due to 'brain disorders'. Nowadays we know that mood disorders are categorised into at least three groups: mixed states, unipolar and bipolar disorder. They usually cause significant handicaps and problems in patients' lives and in many cases lead to disability. In the majority of cases, mood disorders are recurrent and are characterised by many episodes. The duration of each episode varies from several weeks to several months.

Mood disorders are generally characterised by four types of illness episodes: manic, major depressive, hypomanic and mixed states. A patient may have a combination of any of these episodes over the course of the illness. Thus, the presentation of mood disorders can vary widely. Major depression is the most common mood disorder and this has been discussed in Chapter 5. Here we will focus on bipolar mania, but first we need to examine bipolar disorder in more detail.

What is bipolar disorder?

Bipolar disorder is a mood disorder condition that is characterised by alternating periods of depression and mania. There are different types of bipolar disorder but the most common are bipolar I and bipolar II.

Bipolar I patients have full-blown manic episodes or mixed episodes of depression and mania. The course of the illness can be characterised by *rapid cycling*, which means that the patient can suffer at least four episodes in one year. In practice, many patients experience switches in mood more than four times in year. In some patients this rapid cycling manifests as rapid cycling between depressive episodes and mania.

Bipolar II is defined as an illness consisting of one or more major depressive episodes and at least one hypomanic episode.

One of the most important recent developments in the field of mood disorder is the discovery that many patients who appear to be suffering from a major depressive disorder are in fact suffering from a form of bipolar spectrum depression and in particular bipolar II. In the past this has led to many bipolar patients who might have benefited from mood stabiliser and antipsychotic treatment being treated with antidepressant monotherapy, which may increase mood cycling, mixed states and the conversion of hypomania to mania. The case study of Elizabeth above is typical of someone who was treated for unipolar depression, when in fact she was suffering from the depressive phase of a bipolar illness. As much as it is important to distinguish those patients suffering from bipolar spectrum disorder from those suffering from major depression, in reality, patients in the depressive phase of a bipolar illness present with identical symptoms to those suffering from unipolar major depression. To be able to make this distinction, additional information in the form of family history and treatment response is required, as a familial history of bipolar disorder is a strong indicator that the patient has a bipolar spectrum illness, even though the symptoms presented are those of unipolar depression. Patterns of past symptoms can also provide important clues and include previous episodes of hypomania, early age of onset, high frequency of depressive symptoms, high proportion of time unwell, and acute abatement or onset of symptoms.

Current symptom presentation can also provide important clues, for example increased time sleeping, overeating, concurrent anxiety, psychomotor retardation; also, changeable mood, psychotic symptoms and suicidal thoughts can suggest that someone is suffering from bipolar spectrum depression instead of unipolar depression. Therefore, in your interaction with the patient, you need to look out for these symptoms particularly in those whose depression is difficult to treat.

For example, if a patient has been tried on several antidepressants that were not effective, this could be an indication that the patient is suffering from bipolar spectrum depression. Previous responses to antidepressants, such as insomnia, agitation and anxiety, can also be useful in distinguishing bipolar spectrum depression. Again, you need to be watchful of patient response to medication as this can be a useful indicator as to whether a mood stabiliser is indicated or not.

Although these points cannot separate major depression and bipolar spectrum depression with absolute certainty, the point to emphasise here is to exercise vigilance to the possibility that what looks like unipolar depression might in fact be bipolar spectrum depression if investigated more carefully.

As mentioned, bipolar disorder consists of both depressive and manic symptoms. Depressive symptoms have been outlined in Chapter 5, therefore only manic symptoms will be discussed in this chapter before we briefly review common physical disorders and medicines that cause mania. The final sections of the chapter will deal with common treatment errors that should be avoided and what the patient needs to know. Now we turn to bipolar mania.

What is bipolar mania?

Case study

Gale is an 18-year-old A-level student who was admitted to hospital following a summer trip to the USA after her final exams. During her last week on holiday, she was overly talkative and irritable. When she arrived back in the UK, her parents were very concerned about her behaviour, which was out of character. Her parents contacted their GP, who in turn referred Gale to hospital for admission as she was threatening violence. On admission to the ward, she was overly cheerful, overactive, irritable and over-familiar with staff. She talked of being a 'star' and going to Hollywood. She changed clothes very frequently. The night staff reported that she did not sleep at all on her first night. After only two days on the ward, other patients were complaining about her interfering and overbearing manner. She was prescribed haloperidol and lithium carbonate on a regular basis and lorazepam when necessary. After approximately ten days of treatment, her condition started to improve. She was able to reveal that, before she became ill, she was under a great deal of pressure to do well in her A-level exams as she had been offered a conditional place at Cambridge University. She also revealed that her maternal grandmother suffered from bipolar disorder.

Bipolar mania is a state of mind and mood most commonly characterised by excessive energy, along with other symptoms such as extravagant behaviour, rapid speech, reckless spending and, in some instances, psychotic symptoms as in the case study of Gale above. The patient experiences a sustained and abnormally elevated, expansive or irritable mood throughout the episode. The exaggerated mood elevation is beyond what most people would experience and, more than likely, has no relationship to anything going on in the person's life. This is best exemplified by Gale's behaviour during the early stages of admission to hospital.

The manic phase of a bipolar spectrum disorder can be described as *a distinct period of abnormally and persistent elevated expansive or irritable mood lasting at least a week (DSM-IV)*. Manic episodes can be described as mild, moderate or severe. If the condition is described as severe, psychotic symptoms may be present, but not always. Other common symptoms of mania are:

- inflated self-esteem;
- flight of ideas and racing thoughts;
- talkativeness, pressure of speech;
- risk-taking;
- decreased need for sleep;
- increased goal-directed activity;
- behaving inappropriately, for example making crude remarks at a dinner party;
- spending recklessly, such as buying a car without the means to pay for it;
- grandiose thinking, for example believing you are better than anyone else at doing something, or that you can accomplish a difficult task in hours instead of a week;
- hypersexuality, such as making unusual sexual demands of your partner, making inappropriate sexual advances, spending a great deal of money on phone sex, internet pornography or prostitutes, or having affairs;
- dressing and behaving flamboyantly.

Common disorders and medicines that may cause mania

Many mental health disorders can simply be a secondary manifestation of physical illness and therapeutic drugs. The following physical illnesses can present bipolar symptoms:

- neurological disorders such as Huntington's chorea, extrapyramidal disease, Wilson's disease (copper accumulation);
- CNS infections, viral encephalitis;
- cerebral trauma;
- brain tumour;
- cerebral vascular accidents;
- temporal lobe epilepsy
- Pick's disease (chronic constrictive pericarditis);
- hyperthyroidism;
- dialysis dementia;
- pellagra (vitamin B_3 deficiency);
- vitamin B_{12} deficiency;
- post-partum mania;
- influenza;
- multiple sclerosis.

Drugs that can cause bipolar mania are:

- procyclidine
- disulphin
- corticosteroids
- **hallucinogens**

- amphetamines
- bromides
- cocaine
- isoniazid

- procarbazine
- opiates
- cimetidine

The treatment of bipolar spectrum disorders

The treatment of bipolar disorder has at least two important goals: first, the reduction of symptoms and, second, the stabilisation of the illness through medicines and other psychosocial interventions. There is robust evidence to suggest that failure to continue taking medication for this disorder leads to frequent and progressive worsening of symptoms. Subsequent episodes of the illness will become more and more severe and refractory (Gonzalez-Pinto et al., 2010).

Several medicines from different classes of compounds have been used in the treatment of bipolar disorder: during the depressive stage, antidepressants and mood stabilisers are usually the treatment of choice; and in the manic phase, antipsychotics and mood stabilisers. Because antidepressant and antipsychotic therapies are discussed in Chapters 5 and 7 respectively, they will not be covered in this chapter. The following section will discuss the use of mood stabilisers in the treatment of bipolar spectrum disorders.

Mood stabilisers

Mood stabilisers are the main medicines used in the long-term management of bipolar disorder. They are used to maintain a person's mood at a reasonable level and help prevent future episodes of low mood (depression) or high mood (mania). Some are also used to help control episodes of mania. There are several types of mood stabilisers but the oldest medicine is lithium.

Lithium

Lithium has been used in the treatment of bipolar disorder since the nineteenth century, but interest in its use waned for a time before being revived in Australia after the Second World War. Even so, the rest of the world was slow to adopt this treatment, mainly because of deaths that resulted from its use. In the USA, it was not until 1970 that lithium was licensed for the treatment of mania, but only under strict conditions of blood lithium monitoring to reduce the risk of lithium toxicity.

Although lithium has been used to treat bipolar disorder for a long time, it has a complex mode of action that has proved difficult to understand. One popular concept is that it works by altering sodium transport across cell membranes of both nerve and muscle cells. Another theory is that it works by altering the metabolism of neurotransmitters such as serotonin. A third theory is that it works by reducing the responsiveness of neurons to stimuli from muscarinic, cholinergic and alpha$_1$-adrenergic neurotransmitters (see Chapter 4).

Whatever the mode of action of lithium, its effectiveness in people suffering from certain mood disorders is undoubted. It is particularly effective in the treatment and prevention of manic episodes; however, it is less effective in the treatment of bipolar depression. Despite its modest success in the treatment of bipolar depression, it is well established in the prevention of suicide and self-harm. It has been suggested that lithium may not be as effective in the treatment and maintenance of rapid cycling bipolar disorder.

Before a patient starts on lithium, you should explain to them that certain tests need to be carried out, such as kidney function, creatinine clearance, urine specific gravity and thyroid function, as lithium interferes with the regulation of sodium and water levels in the body. In addition, if a patient is above 50 years of age, an ECG should be done before commencement of the medicine, as lithium displaces sodium in the body and this may impact on heart function. The problem becomes more acute with advancing age. As a nurse, you will be responsible for coordinating these tests and you should explain the procedure and reassure the patient.

The dosing of lithium is usually guided by **blood therapeutic drug levels**. During acute treatment, the average daily dose tends to range from 900mg to 2400mg. The blood serum therapeutic levels should be 0.8–1.2mmol/L. During the maintenance phases of the treatment, the average daily dose of the drug should be between 400mg and 1200mg per day. People in the manic stages can have increased tolerance to lithium and therefore may require lithium levels of 0.9–1.4 mmol/L, but this is only in exceptional cases. Before you read further, please try Activity 6.1.

Activity 6.1   *Critical thinking*

A patient is prescribed 400mg lithium carbonate slow-release tablets. During medicines administration, the nurse notices that the slow-release tablets are out of stock and therefore gives the patient two tablets of lithium carbonate each of 200mg.

- Can you explain what the risk is with such an action?

An outline answer is provided at the end of the chapter.

Lithium is completely absorbed in the gastrointestinal tract and peak plasma levels of the medicine occur one and a half to two hours after administration and, if a slow-release preparation is administered, the peak time is increased to four hours. To overcome problems presented by peak plasma levels, a sustained-release formulation should be used. Lithium is excreted mostly through the kidneys and therefore adequate renal function is important, as was mentioned earlier. The blood plasma levels of lithium should be taken seven days after dose initiation and then two-weekly until plasma levels of the drug are stable. If the dose is adjusted, plasma levels of the drug need to be checked. As a nurse, you are responsible for coordinating these tests.

Side effects

Well-known side effects of lithium include gastrointestinal symptoms such as indigestion, nausea and vomiting, and hair loss, weight gain, acne, tremor, sedation, reduced glomerular filtration rate, impaired cognition, weak muscular coordination, excessive urination, abnormal increase in white blood cells, blurred vision, sexual dysfunction and oedema. Excessive lithium retention due to vomiting and diarrhoea can cause lithium toxicity. In this case, the dose of lithium should be lowered. Heavy sweating can also lead to increases in blood lithium levels. Concurrent rapid increase of lithium and an antipsychotic is normally discouraged as this may lead to neurotoxicity.

Special considerations

When lithium is used in the elderly, it is important for you to ensure that the person's kidneys can cope with lithium excretion. This is done by performing a kidney function test. You should also ensure that the person is taking adequate salt and fluid as the ability to excrete lithium decreases with age. This can result in longer elimination time for the medicine. Even at safe therapeutic levels, the elderly are prone to developing cognitive impairment and damage to nervous tissue. Lithium should be started on a relatively lower dose, but you should be aware that side effects can also occur at a relatively lower blood plasma level of the medicine. Slow-release formulations may help to minimise side effects that occur as a result of peak plasma levels. Now try Activity 6.2 before reading further.

Activity 6.2   *Evidence-based practice and research*

Ruth is a 24-year-old woman who has been taking lithium for three years. She informs you that she wishes to start a family, but she is not sure what effect taking lithium will have on her and any potential baby.

• What would your response be?

An outline answer is provided at the end of the chapter.

If at all possible, the use of lithium in pregnant women should be avoided, particularly in the first trimester. Lithium has been associated with increased risk of foetal malformation and premature birth. Its use is also associated with severe infant toxicity, although this has been known to be reversible.

Lithium is also found in the milk of breastfeeding mothers and this causes symptoms such as involuntary movements, dehydration, hypothyroidism, cyanosis, heart murmur and lethargy in the child. If the mother wishes to breastfeed, she should be informed of the risks to the infant while she is taking lithium. The infant's lithium levels and thyroid function should be monitored.

You should take on board that good accurate observation of a patient's behaviour before and after lithium initiation is very important. You should observe for side effects and signs of lithium toxicity and report these immediately, withholding the dose while you inform the doctor. You should closely monitor fluid and particularly salt intake, which should be adjusted if there is any loss of salt through vomiting and diarrhoea. It is important for you to explain to your patient that they should expect generalised discomfort, thirst and frequent urination during the first few days of treatment initiation, but that this will subside within weeks. Your patient should be informed that, to avoid or minimise gastrointestinal disturbance, lithium may be taken with meals. Before you read further, try Activity 6.3.

Activity 6.3 — *Critical thinking*

Steven, a 40-year-old man who is on lithium 1000mg a day, has just informed you that he will not be able to fulfil an appointment scheduled for August because he will be on holiday for two weeks in Cyprus.

- What precautions should Steven take while on holiday?

An outline answer is provided at the end of the chapter.

Management of lithium side effects

The side effects of lithium, and their management, are outlined below.

- **Gastrointestinal problems**: These include indigestion, nausea, vomiting and diarrhoea. These symptoms are common at the initiation of therapy and the dose should be slowly increased. Slow-release preparations can decrease nausea but can increase diarrhoea. Advise the patient to take lithium with meals.
- **Kidney problems**: Unlike many medicines, lithium relies on the kidneys for elimination from the body. Therefore, any slight interference or alteration of the kidneys could lead to a build-up of lithium. Increased thirst (polydipsia) and polyurea (excessive passing of urine) are common side effects. You should encourage the patient to drink a lot of fluids even if experiencing polyurea. Polyurea is common in about 60 per cent of people on long-term treatment. If creatinine increases sharply, the medicine should be withheld until a creatinine tolerance test is done. Alternatively, the lithium dose should be reduced or discontinued altogether. Some patients may experience less polydipsia if the dose of lithium is taken at bedtime.
- **Neurological and cognitive problems**: These include memory impairment, lethargy, weakness, postural tremor and headache. Nearly 50 per cent of patients experience fine hand tremor at some stage during treatment with lithium, but the symptom remits in 90 per cent of cases. Lithium may increase **extrapyramidal side effects (EPS)** in patients taking antipsychotics. In rare cases, it can reactivate neuroleptic malignant syndrome (NMS) (see page 150). The dosage of lithium should be reduced or the interval between doses should be increased. Advise the patient to reduce caffeine and other stimulant use. In some cases, the doctor may prescribe beta-blockers to help reduce tremors. Low doses of lithium should be used in the elderly and those with brain trauma. In some cases, worsening of tremor, confusion, stupor and slurred speech may be signs of lithium toxicity and blood lithium levels

should be taken to rule this out. You should note that, although various methods such as dialysis can be used, there is no antidote for lithium toxicity.

- **Endocrine problems**: Hypothyroidism develops in 20 per cent of patients treated with long-term lithium. Thyroid hormones are usually affected, but in most cases this is not clinically significant. A baseline thyroid function test (TFT) should be done and checked every six months. If thyroid-stimulating hormone (TSH) is elevated, adding thyroxine (T4) should be considered. Baseline calcium and phosphorus should be monitored and this should be followed up every six months.
- **Cardiac problems**: These are mainly minor changes in the ECG. A baseline ECG for those with a history of cardiac problems or over the age of 50 years should be done. If T wave flattening is present, calcium channel blockers and/or beta-blockers should be used. Monitor the pulse periodically and avoid drugs that cause bradyarrythmias.
- **Dermatological problems**: These include acne, hair loss, psoriasis and pruritis. A change in mood stabiliser can be considered if symptoms persist. Anti-acne formulations should be used, but these may be of limited effect.
- **Weight gain**: The increased intake of fluid by patients on lithium may promote weight gain in addition to lithium's insulin-like effect on carbohydrates. Weight gain management should be implemented, avoiding sugary and fatty foods. Medication can be switched to carbamazepine.

Anticonvulsants

Several anticonvulsants have been established as a treatment option in bipolar disorder. They may constitute an alternative to lithium for prophylactic treatment; however, not every anti-convulsant acts as a mood stabiliser. In addition, there are clear differences in their efficacy and tolerability. One of the most commonly used anticonvulsants in the treatment of bipolar illness is sodium valproate, or sodium valproic acid.

Valproic acid

Valproic acid was first made in 1882 and it was mainly used as a solvent until French scientist Pierre Eymard discovered its anticonvulsant properties. Valproic acid has been increasingly used in the treatment of bipolar disorder but, as with most anticonvulsants, its mode of action is not clear. One popular theory is that valproic acid works by reducing the level of excitation of neurons. It does this by reducing the flow of sodium into the nerve cell through sodium channels. It has also been postulated that it works by interfering with calcium channels and indirectly blocks glutamate action. A third theory is that this medicine increases the concentration of GABA (see Chapter 4) by a mechanism that is yet to be uncovered.

Research evidence seems to suggest that valproic acid is effective in the treatment of bipolar disorder (Bond et al., 2010). In particular, it is effective in the treatment of mania, in mixed states or for patients with secondary or rapid cycling disorder. Oral valproic acid can lead to rapid stabilisation of manic symptoms. The medicine can take anything from a few days to a few months to stabilise a bipolar condition.

Before valproic acid treatment, blood platelet levels, coagulation tests and a liver function test should be done. It is your responsibility as the nurse to coordinate these tests within the multi-disciplinary team. During the first few months of treatment with valproic acid, liver function tests and platelet counts are monitored regularly and again the nurse has a lead role in coordinating these. Once the condition has stabilised, then the tests can be reduced to twice a year. Like lithium, valproic acid is associated with weight gain (Bond et al., 2010) and, therefore, you should monitor the patient's weight closely. If your patient is already overweight, with a body mass index (BMI) above or equal to 25, a pre-diabetes test (fasting blood glucose) should be performed. If the test is positive, you should refer the patient for weight management or nutritional advice to a specialist, usually a dietician. If a patient on valproic acid gains more than 5 per cent of initial weight, you should bring this to the attention of the doctor so that a pre-diabetes or **dys-lipidaemia** test can be done. Usually, valproic acid can be started at doses of 250mg per day and gradually increased until therapeutic levels are reached or until side effects become intolerable. The dose range for valproic acid is between 750mg and 3000mg per day in single or divided dose. The recommended plasma level for valproic acid is 350–800µmol/L.

Side effects

Common side effects of valproic acid are indigestion and/or weight gain. Less common are fatigue, swelling of tissues, usually in the lower limbs, acne, dizziness, drowsiness, hair loss, headaches, nausea, sedation and tremors. Valproic acid levels within the normal range are capable of causing excess of ammonia in the blood, or hyperammonaemia, which can lead to brain damage. Rarely, valproic acid can cause blood abnormality, impaired liver function, jaundice, an abnormally small number of platelets in the blood (thrombocytopenia), and prolonged coagulation times. In about 5 per cent of pregnant women, valproic acid will cross the placenta and cause congenital anomalies. Due to these side effects, most doctors will ask for blood tests, initially and then as often as once a week, reducing to once every two months. Temporary liver enzyme increase has been reported in 20 per cent of cases during the first few months of taking this medicine. Inflammation of the liver (hepatitis), the first symptom of which is jaundice, is found in rare cases.

There have also been reports of **cognitive dysfunction**, Parkinsonian symptoms, and even reversible shrinkage (pseudoatrophy) of the brain in long-term treatment with valproic acid.

Special considerations

If possible, the use of valproic acid should be avoided in pregnant women because of the incidence of baby malformation, which can be as much as 11 per cent. The serum levels of babies are likely to be higher than those of expectant mothers and the half-life of the medicine in the infant is likely to be longer than that of the mother, presenting considerable health problems for the infant. Some of the problems for babies associated with maternal use of valproic acid are spina bifida risk, neural tube defects, neurological dysfunction and general developmental deficits, which can involve as many as 70 per cent of children. Infants may be at a relatively higher risk of hypoglycaemia.

No clear evidence of valproic acid harm has been seen in breastfeeding mothers, even though the half-life of the drug is higher for the baby than the mother. You should inform parents of the possible risk of liver impairment and blood abnormalities in the infant. Also, liver enzymes of both the mother and the infant should be monitored.

Management of valproic acid side effects

The most common side effects of valproic acid are gastrointestinal problems and weight gain. For the management of these, please see under 'Management of lithium side effects' (pages 126–7).

Carbamazepine

Carbamazepine was first discovered in Switzerland by the scientist Walter Schindler and was initially used to treat **trigeminal neuralgia**. It has been available in the UK as an anti-convulsant since 1965, but its use as a mood stabiliser started in Japan in the 1970s. Unlike lithium and valproic acid, the mechanism of action of carbamazepine is fairly well understood. It works by blocking sodium channels, therefore making nerve cells (neurons) less excitable. Furthermore, it has been hypothesised that it also works by blocking calcium and potassium ion channels, potentiating the inhibitory effects of GABA (see Chapter 4).

Carbamazepine is effective in the treatment of manic symptoms, rapid cycling and mixed bipolar states, and it normally takes a few weeks for effects to be noticed. Overall, it is as effective as valproic acid and lithium in the treatment of manic symptoms; however, there is some evidence to suggest that carbamazepine is more effective in major depressive disorder.

Before a patient can be commenced on carbamazepine, you should ensure that blood count, liver and kidney function and thyroid function tests are done. After the initiation of treatment you should ensure that a blood count is done every two to four weeks for the first two months. This can be reduced to every three to six months throughout the treatment. With respect to kidney, thyroid and liver functions, you should ensure that these tests are done every six to twelve months. The recommended plasma level for carbamazepine is 17–54μmol/L.

In bipolar disorder, initial doses should be 400mg daily and the dose can be increased by 200mg per week, usually in divided doses. In acute conditions, the daily dose can be as high as 1200mg, and in maintenance doses it can be between 800mg and 1200mg per day. Please note that, if carbamazepine liquid suspension is to be administered, it reaches a higher blood serum peak level than the same dose of the tablet form; for this reason, carbamazepine suspension formulation should be started at a lower dose and then titrated up slowly. The downside of slow titration is that it delays therapeutic effects. Controlled-release formulations can significantly reduce side effects and carbamazepine should be slowly titrated when the patient is taking other sedating medicines or anticonvulsants.

Side effects

The side effects due to carbamazepine are caused by excessive action of the drug on the sodium channels and include sedation, dizziness, confusion, unsteadiness, headache, nausea, vomiting, diarrhoea, dry mouth, blurred vision, menstrual disturbances, weight gain and skin rash. Carbamazepine also presents with rare but life-threatening side effects such as **aplastic anaemia**, **agranulocytosis**, cardiac problems, and activation of suicidal ideation and behaviour. It can also cause a rare but severe dermatological condition called *Stevens–Johnson syndrome*. Stevens–Johnson syndrome is a life-threatening condition affecting the skin in which cell death causes the epidermis to separate from the dermis.

Special considerations

Because the medicine is excreted by the kidneys, the dose of carbamazepine is normally lowered in those with kidney impairment. Also, the medicine should be used with care for those who have liver impairment, as cases of liver failure have been reported. The use of carbamazepine in those with cardiac problems is normally restricted.

Like lithium and valproic acid, the use of carbamazepine in pregnancy should be restricted because of reported incidences of foetal malformation. If carbamezapine is to be given to someone pregnant, blood serum levels of the medicine should be monitored throughout the pregnancy. The medicine can cause birth abnormalities and vitamin K deficiency. In breastfeeding, the drug serum levels should be monitored in the infant, and the mother should be informed about the signs and symptoms of liver dysfunction.

Management of common carbamazepine side effects

Many of the side effect management issues are the same as with antidepressants (Chapter 5) and antipsychotics (Chapter 7). Side effects not covered there are listed below.

- **Neurological side effects**: These are usually temporary, but a dose reduction can sometimes help. See Chapter 7 on the management of antipsychotic side effects.
- **Leucopenia**: This is a decrease in the number of white blood cells in the body. It is usually temporary but, if it persists, the dose of carbamazepine can be reduced.
- **Skin rash**: Advise the patient to use topical steroids. If the rash is accompanied by fever, skin lesions and bleeding, this could be an indication of Stevens–Johnson syndrome; the drug should be discontinued and the doctor informed immediately.
- **Hypnotraemia**: This is a disturbance of the salts in the blood. Carbamazepine should be discontinued if the condition is severe.
- **Liver enzyme elevation**: This is usually benign but doses can be reduced if it persists. Clinical status should be monitored to rule out general discomfort, jaundice and vomiting.
- **Thyroid dysfunction**: A slight elevation of free T4 is usually benign, but a thyroid supplement should be considered if TSH is high.

Lamotrigine

Since 1994, lamotrigine has been used to treat partial seizures in epilepsy. It was not until 2003 that this medicine was used as a mood stabiliser in bipolar disorder. Like most mood stabilisers, the mode of action of lamotrigine is poorly understood. Laboratory pharmacological studies suggest that lamotrigine has been shown to inhibit sodium channels and thereby inhibit the release of excitatory neurotransmitters such as glutamate. One interesting thing about lamotrigine is that, while a majority of mood stabilisers work mostly by controlling the manic phase of bipolar disorder, lamotrigine tends to be most effective in the treatment and prophylaxis of bipolar depression. Most importantly, it treats bipolar depression without triggering mania, hypomania, mixed states or rapid cycling. To date, there is little evidence for its efficacy in the treatment of the manic phase of the disorder. It is recommended as the first-line treatment for acute depression in bipolar depression as well as the maintenance. If lamotrigine is given at **sub-therapeutic** dose, it has a mild antidepressant effect.

Currently, there is no need to monitor blood plasma before commencing lamotrigine. Generally, the medicine should be initiated at very low doses to minimise the incidence of skin rash (see 'Side effects' below). The starting dose is usually 25mg/day for the first two weeks. This can be increased to 50mg/day for a further three weeks. From week five, the medicine can be increased to 100mg/day and then increased to 200mg/day (maximum dose) at week six. If the patient stops taking lamotrigine for five days or more, the best course of action may be to restart the drug with initial dose titration to minimise the incidence of skin rash. Also, patients should not be started on lamotrigine within two weeks of a viral infection, skin rash or vaccination.

Side effects

Common side effects include headaches, dizziness and insomnia. Others include acne and skin irritation (as mentioned above), vivid dreams or nightmares, night sweats, body aches and cramps, muscle aches, dry mouth, mouth ulcers, damage to tooth enamel, fatigue, memory and cognitive problems, irritability, weight changes, hair loss, changes in libido, frequent urination, nausea, appetite changes. In very rare cases, lamotrigine has been known to cause Stevens–Johnson syndrome (see page 130).

Special considerations

Unlike most other anticonvulsants, women are more likely than men to have side effects of lamotrigine. This may be due to interaction between lamotrigine and female hormones. It is of particular concern for women on oestrogen-containing hormonal contraceptives, which have been shown to decrease blood serum levels of lamotrigine (see Chapter 11). Women starting an oestrogen-based oral contraceptive may need to increase the dosage of lamotrigine to maintain its level of efficacy. Similarly, women may experience an increase in lamotrigine side effects upon discontinuation of a contraceptive. This may include the 'pill-free' week, where lamotrigine serum levels have been shown to increase twofold. There is a significant increase in **follicle-stimulating hormone (FSH)** and **luteinising hormone (LH)** in women taking lamotrigine with oral contraceptives, compared to women taking oral contraceptives alone.

The use of lamotrigine in pregnancy is normally restricted and should be used if its potential benefits clearly outweigh the risks, as there is tentative evidence that it may cause cleft palate in babies. Lamotrigine is excreted in breast milk and therefore breastfeeding is not normally recommended during treatment. Infant serum levels can be between 25 and 30 per cent of those of the mother and this risks life-threatening rash in the baby. Lamotrigine can inhibit sleep, so the medicine is best taken in the morning. Before you read further, try Activity 6.4.

For the management of common lamotrigine side effects, see that outlined above for carbamazepine, lithium and sodium valproic acid.

Atypical antipsychotics

In the past, typical as well as atypical antipsychotics have been used as adjunct treatments for bipolar disorder, but there is emerging evidence for the monotherapy use of these medicines as mood stabilisers. Olanzapine and quetiapine have been mostly used in the treatment of bipolar disorder, but other antipsychotics such as risperidone, zisprasidone, aripiprazole and clozapine have also been used. Usually, the severity of the symptoms, as well as the side effects profile of the antipsychotic, are determining factors in choosing the right antipsychotic. In particular, where a patient is suffering from psychotic symptoms such as delusions and hallucinations, antipsychotics are indicated. For antipsychotic modes of action, side effects and their management, please refer to Chapter 7.

Common treatment errors to avoid

Lithium is very toxic and close monitoring is required particularly for those patients who are suicidal. Suicidal ideation should be monitored even in those suffering from the manic phase of the disorder. Dehydration can be a problem, particularly in manic patients who may be overactive and therefore you should encourage adequate fluid intake. In general, people with bipolar illness require lifelong treatment. Discontinuation of mood stabilisers will often result in relapse that is even more severe. If discontinuation must be undertaken, the medicine should be gradually withdrawn over a period of six weeks. Sustained-release medication should never be crushed as this will result in rapid absorption causing toxic symptoms.

What the patient needs to know

- Lithium, valproic acid, carbamazepine, lamotrigine and other medicines such as olanzapine and quetiapine are drugs that will treat mood or emotional problems. They also help with preventing relapse. It is important to take these medicines and follow instructions as prescribed.

- Mood stabilisers such as lithium, valproic acid, lamotrigine and carbamazepine are not addictive.
- Many side effects of mood stabilisers can be minimised by taking the medicines in divided doses.
- Because the therapeutic and toxic dosage of lithium are so close to each other, regular blood tests will be performed to ensure that blood lithium levels are within the therapeutic range only.
- Bipolar disorder is biological, not a moral defect or character flaw. It is a treatable illness that runs in families. When severe, the patient may not always be able to control behaviour.
- Patients taking lithium should be warned not to take over-the-counter non-steroidal anti-inflammatory drugs (NSAIDs) such as ibuprofen. Prescribing NSAIDs for such patients should be avoided if possible, and if they are prescribed the patient should be closely monitored.
- Anticonvulsant mood stabilisers can cause birth defects, so if the patient is planning to have a family, she should contact the prescriber for more advice.
- Lifestyle changes that promote both physical and mental health should be discussed with the patient. These include the avoidance of sleep deprivation, even for one night, and avoidance of shift work, alcohol, illicit drugs, and other substances that interfere with sleep such as caffeine and decongestants.
- Decreased exposure to light, particular in winter, can trigger bipolar depression and excessive exposure to sunlight, particularly in summer, can trigger mania.
- There are many self-help groups that provide support for bipolar patients and their families. You should provide information on these and other relevant organisations within the patient's area.

Chapter summary

Bipolar illness belongs to a group of mood disorders that are typically a mixture of depressive and manic phases. During the depressive phase of the illness, the patient may present with typical symptoms of major depressive disorder such as a low mood, apathy, poor concentration, appetite and sleep, cognitive changes and suicidal ideation. In the manic phase of the illness, the patient typically presents with a euphoric mood that is not matched by the patient's circumstances. Other symptoms may include irritability, grandiosity, racing thoughts, delusions and hallucinations.

Subtle differences between unipolar and bipolar depression exist. Bipolar depression tends to occur at a younger age and is almost sudden in onset. Also, recovery from bipolar depression can be spontaneous and patients can go into a manic phase after recovery from depression. Mood stabilisers are a group of medicines that prevent the patient from having extremes of mood (depressed or manic). Most commonly used mood stabilisers are lithium, sodium valproic acid, carbamazepine and lamotrigine.

Activities: brief outline answers

Activity 6.1 Lithium carbonate dosage error (page 124)

Slow-release medicine is designed so that a small amount of the medicine is released into the blood to avoid toxic levels. Therefore, if ordinary lithium tablets are administered in high doses, they will be absorbed very quickly into the blood stream, thus elevating blood serum levels and risking lithium toxicity.

Activity 6.2 Lithium and pregnancy (page 125)

Lithium, like most mood stabilisers, should be avoided in pregnancy because there is a high risk of foetal malformation and premature birth. Inform Ruth about this risk; it may be that Ruth will need to reduce the dose of lithium or stop altogether should she become pregnant.

Activity 6.3 Lithium use on holiday (page 126)

As Steven is going to Cyprus in August, the weather is likely to be hot and therefore he is likely to sweat a lot. In turn, this is likely to raise his blood lithium to toxic levels. He should be advised to drink lots of water. Alternatively, and more appropriately, you should ask the prescriber to review his lithium with a view to reducing the dose for the period he is on holiday.

Activity 6.4 Lamotrigine side effects (page 132)

You should advise Charles not to take any more lamotrigine until it's confirmed that the skin rash and lesions are not due to lamotrigine side effects. You should contact the prescriber as well as his GP without delay.

Further reading

Preston, JD, O'Neal, JH and Talaga, MC (2008) *A Handbook of Clinical Psychopharmacology*, 5th edition. Oakland, CA: New Harbinger Publications.

A clearly written book and particularly useful for those from a non-medical background. It explains non-pharmacological mental healthcare well.

Stahl, SM (2009) *Stahl's Essential Psychopharmacology: The prescriber's guide*, 3rd edition. Cambridge: Cambridge University Press.

A comprehensive guide to psychopharmacology that is clearly written and has good illustrations.

Taylor, D, Paton, C and Kapur, S (2009) *The Maudsley Prescribing Guidelines*, 10th edition. London: Informa Healthcare.

A very useful, easy-to-understand, evidence-based prescribing and general medicines management manual. It is particularly useful for prescribers.

Useful websites

www.drugs.com

This website provides a lot of useful information that ranges from pill identification to different types of medicines and their interactions, and new medicines on the market.

www.medicines.org.uk/emc

This website explains all drug actions, side effects and interactions. It is a very good reference source, particularly for those who prescribe medicines.

www.mhf.org.uk/information/mental-health-a-z

The Mental Health Foundation offers information and publications to download on research, good practice in services, and mental health problems and key issues. It provides a daily mental health news service and directories of organisations, websites and events.

Chapter 7
Management and treatment
of psychotic disorders

Introduction

The word 'psychosis' comes from the Greek and literally means an abnormal condition of the mind. Over the centuries, stigma and fear have surrounded the idea of psychosis and a good example of this is its use in such everyday phrases as 'psychotic rage' and 'psychotic killers'. It is therefore not surprising that the treatment and care of people with psychosis provoke lively debates; no other psychiatric illness evokes so much controversy, emotion and misunderstanding. Because of the stigma surrounding this illness, you are advised to consult a specialist textbook and learn as much about this illness as you can.

An important aspect of psychosis is that there are many ways in which the illness presents itself. Because of this, symptoms of psychosis tend to vary, although the medicines used to treat psychotic illnesses are the same regardless of the form of the psychosis. Most textbooks of psychiatry divide psychosis into three categories: schizophrenia; psychotic mood disorders; and psychosis associated with neurological disorders. *Schizophrenia* is probably the most talked and written about of all psychotic illnesses. For this reason, we will confine ourselves to talking about schizophrenia and its treatment.

The term 'schizophrenia' is less than 100 years old. Neurologist Emil Kraepelin first identified the disease as a separate mental illness in 1887. Written documents that identify schizophrenia can be traced back to ancient Egypt, as far back as the second millennium BC. Depression, dementia and thought disturbances that are typical of schizophrenia are described in detail in the Ebers Papyrus, or the Book of Hearts: the heart and the mind seem to have been synonymous in ancient Egypt (Joachim, 1890).

The public health importance of schizophrenia is clear. Nearly 0.1 per cent of any population suffers from this serious illness and it starts from adolescence to early adulthood. As in psychosis in general, the symptoms of schizophrenia are many and diverse but can be broadly divided into five syndromes: positive, negative, disorganisation, affective and cognitive. For a more a comprehensive coverage of these syndromes you are advised to consult a specialist book on schizophrenia and its symptoms.

This chapter provides an overview of the treatment of psychosis and it will begin by outlining the physical illness and medicines that may cause psychosis. This should encourage you to think of psychosis as an illness that is a result of a complex interplay of social, psychological and biological stressors. The chapter then explores the dopamine theory of psychosis as a way of providing you with the necessary background knowledge into understanding the mechanism of action of antipsychotic medicines. The difference between conventional antipsychotics and 'atypicals' will be explored before common side effects are covered. The final sections of the chapter will deal with how you can advise patients to manage different types of side effects, errors to avoid during treatment and what the patient needs to know.

Physical diseases that may cause psychosis

The psychosis that can result from non-psychological conditions is sometimes known as *secondary psychosis* and certain physical illnesses have been known to cause this. It is important for you to be aware of your patient's full medical history as this is a prerequisite to good clinical decision-making. If a patient's psychotic symptoms are due to a physical disorder, it is preferable and more effective to treat the underlying physical illness first.

Case study

A 45-year-old man with a history of alcohol dependence and sleeping rough was found wandering the streets in the early hours of the morning. He was not intoxicated but was confused and could not remember where he was; he gave his name as Neil and could not elaborate further. The police noticed that he was talking to himself a lot and trying to 'pick up things' from the floor that were not there. Also, he kept scratching his skin and complained of insects crawling all over his body. He was brought to hospital under the terms of the Mental Health Act. He refused to go to bed for fear of ghosts and he could see spiders on the floor. As his condition was unknown, the team decided to monitor his condition without administering medication for at least a week. However, the team noticed that he was emaciated and this suggested that his dietary intake before admission to hospital was poor. He was prescribed some vitamin supplements and part of the care plan was 'to encourage adequate fluid and dietary intake'. Neil's condition gradually improved and he was able to give his full name and address and name the hospitals he had been admitted to for alcohol detoxification.

Some of the physical illnesses that can cause secondary psychosis are:

- Addison's disease
- Cushing's syndrome
- brain injury
- vitamin deficiency: folic acid (B_{12})
- toxic states (delirium)
- Huntington's chorea or disorder (HD)
- dementia with Lewy bodies (DLB)
- multiple sclerosis

- myxoedema
- pancreatitis
- pellagra
- pernicious anaemia
- porphyria
- thyrotoxicosis
- temporal lobe epilepsy

Activity 7.1   *Critical thinking*

You notice that a doctor has taken a blood sample for biochemistry analysis from a 68-year-old lady who lives alone; she has recently been admitted to your ward. She looks emaciated, disoriented and restless. The doctor has written in her notes 'For electrolytes test'.

- What is the importance of testing for electrolytes in the elderly?

An outline answer is provided at the end of the chapter.

In summary, the physical conditions that can cause psychosis are many and diverse; therefore, it is important to be vigilant as to a patient's physical state as this can provide an important explanation of their mental state. A correct and thorough assessment of the patient's problems is the first important step towards correct treatment that will ultimately lead to good recovery. Now that you understanding how some physical illnesses can cause secondary psychosis, try Activity 7.2.

Activity 7.2   *Critical thinking*

A patient was admitted two weeks ago suffering from a psychotic illness; she is restless, thought disordered and has difficulty sleeping. During a conversation, she informs you that her mother died from cancer of the thyroid but she did not disclose this information to the doctor because she did not think it was relevant.

- Would you recommend a physical health test, and if so which one and why?

An outline answer is provided at the end of the chapter.

Medicines that may cause psychosis

Certain medications, chemicals, toxins or substances may cause psychotic illnesses, so it is important for you to understand the different medicines used in clinical practice that can cause psychotic symptoms. An important part of medicines management is for you to have a good understanding of physical medicines that your patient is taking. This will give you a more rounded view of your patient's problems that will inform your decision-making.

Activity 7.3   *Decision-making*

You have been asked to complete admission procedures for a 19-year-old man who has been brought to your ward. He has no previous history of psychiatric illness but has recently been to Amsterdam with his friends. He has agreed to provide a urine sample for routine examination.

- What might you include in the screening process?

An outline answer is provided at the end of the chapter.

Some substances and medications that may cause psychotic illnesses are:

- L-dopa;
- hallucinogenic substances;
- anticholinergic medicines;

- anti-inflammatory medicines;
- CNS stimulants (psychostimulants).

How psychotic symptoms arise

To be able to understand how antipsychotics work, it is important to begin by determining how psychotic symptoms arise in the first place. A comprehensive coverage of psychopathology is beyond the scope of this book and you should consult a specialist textbook on the subject. However, this section will briefly discuss commonly accepted theories of the mechanism of psychosis.

Psychosis, like many mental health disorders, is thought to be the result of an interaction between a person's intrinsic biological factors and the stress they experience in life. This viewpoint is best explained by the *stress vulnerability model* (Zubin and Spring, 1977), which suggests that people become ill when the stress they face becomes more than they can cope with. Also, people's ability to deal with stress, that is, their vulnerability, differs from person to person: a problem that one person may take in their stride might be enough to cause another person to become depressed or psychotic. In psychosis, the symptoms are accompanied by biological changes, which include abnormal levels of dopamine in various dopamine pathways in the brain (see Figure 7.1). In the mesolimbic pathway there are increased dopamine levels and in the mesocortical pathway there are reduced levels. This observation gave rise to the *dopamine theory*, proposed by Carlsson and Lindqvist in 1963.

The dopamine theory proposes that there is an abnormal increase of dopamine neurotransmission in critical neural pathways in the brain in someone experiencing a psychotic illness. In recent years, neuroimaging techniques have been used to examine brain dopamine function in people with schizophrenia and have supported this hypothesis.

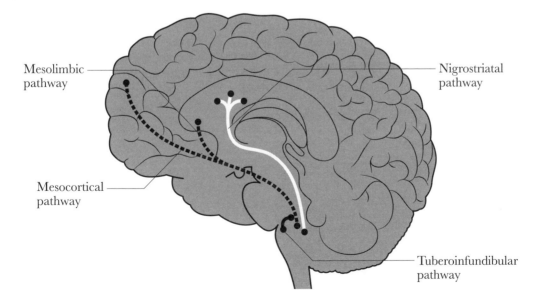

Mesolimbic pathway

Nigrostriatal pathway

Mesocortical pathway

Tuberoinfundibular pathway

Figure 7.1: The four main dopamine pathways

In summary, the dopamine theory in its simplest form suggests that symptoms of schizophrenia are due to an imbalance of dopamine in critical dopamine pathways in the brain (see Figure 7.2). In the mesolimbic pathway, there is too much dopamine entering the synapse. This 'overload' causes the receptors in this region to become overexcited or overstimulated, resulting in information being abnormally processed (see Figure 7.3). This abnormal processing of information leads to positive symptoms such as delusions, hallucinations, thought disorder and bizarre behaviour. In contrast, it is believed that negative symptoms such lack of motivation, lack of ability to enjoy things in life and cognitive symptoms such as poor memory and poor ability to plan or carry out a task are caused by a different mechanism (Featherstone et al., 2007).

Negative and cognitive symptoms are thought to result from too little dopamine in the mesocortical region of the brain (hypodopaminergia) resulting in understimulation (hypoactivation) of post-synaptic dopamine receptors (see Figure 7.4). The understimulation of dopamine receptors in the mesocortical region will cause an abnormal processing of information leading to negative, cognitive and mood (affective) symptoms.

How antipsychotics work

The discovery of the medicines that can effectively treat psychoses (primarily schizophrenia) began in the 1940s. A French surgeon, Henri Laborit, convinced that many of the deaths associated with surgery could be attributed to a patient's fears, found the sedatives promethazine and chlorpromazine, both of which proved to be dramatically effective. The use of chlorpromazine spread to the psychiatric clinic in the mid-1950s, and was found to produce not only

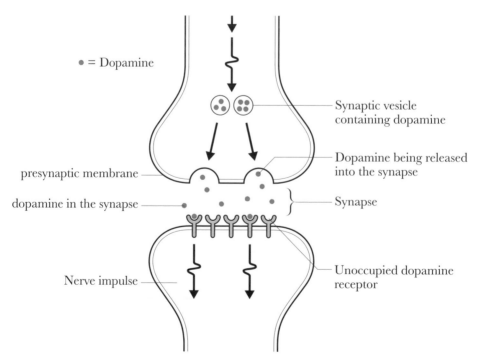

Figure 7.2: Normal dopamine release into the synapse

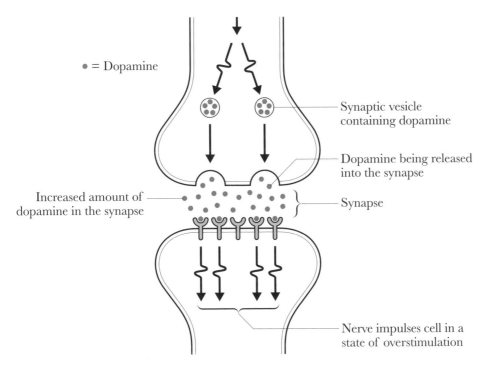

Figure 7.3: An elevated release of dopamine into the synapse, or hyperdopaminergia, resulting in positive symptoms of psychosis

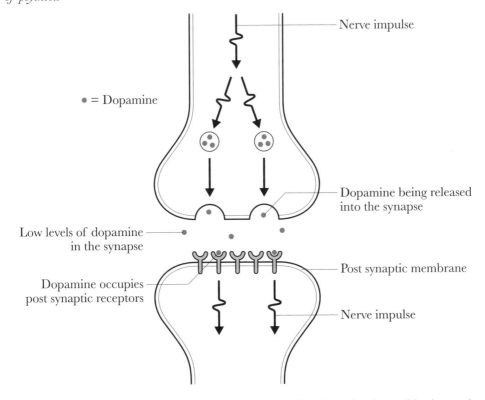

Figure 7.4: Low levels of dopamine release in the synapse, or hypodopaminergia, resulting in negative, cognitive and mood symptoms

sedation but also an equally dramatic reversal of the psychotic symptoms of schizophrenia. Chlorpromazine causes slowness of motor function or 'neurolepsis', emotional blunting or indifference in mood. Chlorpromazine and other early medicines belong to a class of medicines we generally call conventional antipsychotics.

Conventional antipsychotics

As previously mentioned, positive symptoms of psychosis are due to too much dopamine being released into the synapse resulting in overstimulation of the post-synaptic dopamine receptors in the mesolimbic region. All antipsychotics work by blocking or *antagonising* these receptors. When a receptor is antagonised, it can no longer transmit impulses or 'messages' and this reverses the effects of hyperactivation (see Figure 7.5).

Unfortunately, apart from blocking dopamine receptors in the mesolimbic region, antipsychotics also block dopamine receptors in the mesocortical region, an area that suffers from too little dopamine in people with schizophrenia (hypoactivity). Antipsychotic action in this region worsens negative mood and cognitive symptoms. The challenge therefore is to find a medicine that can reduce hyperactivity of dopamine in the mesolimbic region and improve hypoactivity in the mesocortical regions at the same time. In other words, we need to find a medicine that can effectively treat positive as well as negative symptoms. To some degree, the atypical antipsychotics partially meet this challenge and will be discussed next. But before you read further, try Activity 7.4.

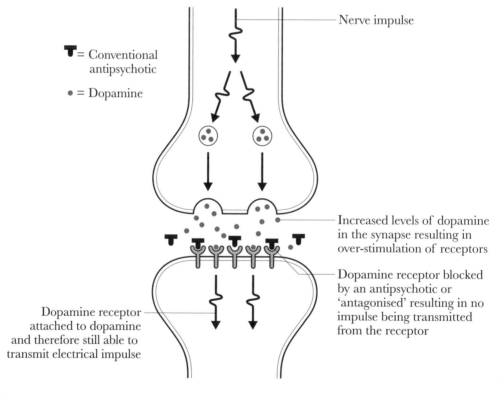

Figure 7.5: Post-synaptic dopamine receptors antagonised by antipsychotics, reversing the effects of overstimulation by dopamine

> **Activity 7.4**   *Critical thinking*
>
> A 46-year old-woman with a long history of being involved with mental health services was readmitted to your ward four days ago. She believes her neighbours have been spying on her using CCTV cameras planted in her house. She spends most of the time sleeping in bed. She has been prescribed and is taking haloperidol 20mg per day.
>
> - What concerns do you have about this woman taking haloperidol?
> - How would you improve the situation?
>
> *An outline answer is provided at the end of the chapter.*

What makes a medicine atypical?

Older conventional antipsychotics such as haloperidol are effective in treating positive symptoms of psychosis but they cause other problems such as worsening of negative symptoms. They also cause side effects such as extrapyramidal side effects (EPS) through their blockade of the nigrostriatal dopamine pathway. EPS are neurologically based body movement disorders that resemble those seen in **idiopathic** Parkinsonism. The mechanism underlying EPS will be explained in later sections.

Atypical antipsychotics have a low tendency to cause EPS and are effective at improving negative symptoms. From a pharmacological point of view, an atypical antipsychotic may mean (1) a medicine that blocks both dopamine and serotonin receptors and (2) a medicine that antagonises dopamine but can dissociate from the receptors very quickly compared to conventional antipsychotics. These medicines are now widely used in clinical practice.

Apart from blocking dopamine D_2 receptors, almost all atypical antipsychotics block serotonin receptors as well (mainly $5HT_2$, $5HT_1$), which serves two functions, depending on the region of the brain: stimulating the release of dopamine into the synapse, and slowing down the release of dopamine in the synapse.

As mentioned previously, negative, cognitive and mood symptoms are the result of too little dopamine in the mesocortical regions of the brain (hypoactivity) and administering conventional antipsychotics is likely to worsen these symptoms. The patient may benefit from atypical antipsychotic medicines.

Let us look at serotonin's involvement in mesocortical dopamine. Serotonin receptors are found on dopamine pathway neurons and some of these receptors are found presynaptically. When serotonin binds to these presynaptic receptors, it inhibits the release of dopamine into the synapse. However, the blockade of presynaptic serotonin receptors by an atypical antipsychotic (atypical antipsychotics block dopamine and serotonin receptors) has the effect of releasing more dopamine into the synapse, thus improving negative, cognitive and mood symptoms. Theoretically, this explains why atypical antipsychotics are better at treating negative, cognitive and affective symptoms compared to conventional antipsychotics.

One of the disadvantages of antipsychotics is that they block receptors in non-therapeutic pathways, such as the nigrostriatal and tuberoinfundibular pathways. The *nigrostriatal pathway* is one of the four major dopamine pathways in the brain (see Figure 7.1 on page 139) and is particularly involved in the regulation of body movement; it is part of a system called the **basal ganglia motor loop**. In schizophrenia, dopamine output in the nigrostriatal pathway is normal, but D_2 receptor blockade by antipsychotics causes the aforementioned extrapyramidal side effects (EPS) – a variety of movement and coordination-related side effects. This is particularly the case if conventional antipsychotics such as haloperidol are used. If atypical antipsychotics such as olanzapine are used, the situation is slightly different.

Antipsychotics also act on a fourth dopamine pathway called the *tuberoinfundibular pathway* (see Figure 7.1 on page 139). This pathway runs between the hypothalamus and the pituitary gland and dopamine levels in this pathway are normal in people with schizophrenia. Blocking dopamine receptors in this region causes sexual and hormonal side effects such as increased levels of prolactin, disruptions to the menstrual cycle in women, visual problems, headache and sexual dysfunction.

If patients use conventional antipsychotics, blocking D_2 receptors in the tuberoinfundibular region causes sexual side effects and increases the flow of prolactin into the blood. The situation is slightly different if atypical antipsychotics are used; while the blockade of dopamine receptors stimulates the release of prolactin, the blockade of serotonin receptors inhibits the release of prolactin, thus counteracting the effect of dopamine blockade. This opposing and simultaneous effect of dopamine and serotonin blockade results in normal levels of prolactin when an atypical medicine is administered. In theory, an antipsychotic's ability to keep prolactin at normal levels is another definition of atypicality. Before proceeding further, please try Activity 7.5.

Activity 7.5   *Critical thinking*

Which of these medicines would you expect to cause sexual dysfunction in patients?

- Haloperidol   • Olanzapine   • Quetiapine

An outline answer is provided at the end of the chapter.

Common antipsychotic side effects

Although antipsychotics do not provide a permanent cure for psychosis, they play an important role during treatment and recovery; their beneficial effects have been established beyond doubt. Cunningham Owens (1999) has asserted that these medicines have played an important role in reversing centuries-old misconceptions of psychosis, both lay and professional; they have also made it possible to implement humane models of care for some of the most vulnerable and misunderstood people.

Like all medicines, antipsychotics come as part of a package that includes therapeutic and non-therapeutic effects. The adverse side effects can be broadly divided into two groups: extrapyramidal side effects (EPS) and non-extrapyramidal side effects.

The non-extrapyramidal side effects are due to antipsychotic medication's action on other systems in the brain, such as their blockade of the histamine, muscarinic and alpha-adrenergic receptors and the tuberoinfundibular pathway. The following section will discuss the commonly experienced side effects in more detail.

Extrapyramidal side effects

PET studies of dopamine have found that antipsychotic blockade of nigrostriatal D_2 sites is related to EPS. The likelihood of EPS development is highest when more than 80 per cent of D_2 receptors in this region are antagonised. At clinically effective doses, some of the newer atypical antipsychotic medicines block less than 80 per cent of D_2 receptors, which may partly explain their clinical efficacy with minimal side effects. EPS can take several forms, including dystonia, akathisia, pseudo-Parkinsonism and tardive dyskinesia and we will look at these next.

Dystonia

Dystonia refers to an abnormality of voluntary muscle tone. It is characterised by involuntary contraction or spasm of the muscles, most commonly affecting the head and neck, which can be painful and frightening. For example, the jaw may be forced to open, which can result in dislocation. Laryngeal spasms can be life-threatening. About 10 per cent of all patients taking conventional antipsychotics experience dystonia as an adverse effect, typically within hours of initiating treatment. They are most common with intramuscular injections of high-potency antipsychotics and in young men below the age of 40. For those who are at high risk of the condition, prophylactic treatment with anticholinergic medication such as procyclidine is generally recommended.

Activity 7.6   *Critical thinking*

Dave is a 23-year-old man who has been admitted to hospital following attempted suicide. He had been troubled for some time by hearing a 'voice of the devil' and bad people saying derogatory things about him. He was prescribed trifluperazine 15mg a day. After three days, his condition deteriorated, and he was more restless, irritable and at times aggressive.

*   In your care plan review, what issues are you likely to consider?

An outline answer is provided at the end of the chapter.

Akathisia

Akathisia is a subjective feeling of muscular discomfort and inner restlessness; a compulsion to move the legs when sitting and an inability to stand still in one place are the most commonly observed features. About 25 per cent of patients treated with conventional antipsychotics will develop akathisia. This symptom is probably the most disabling and intolerable side effect that develops early during the treatment process. Akathisia, which can resemble psychotic agitation, is often associated with higher doses of medication and may be found in tandem with other EPS.

Women are twice as likely as men to experience akathisia. All classes of antipsychotic are known to cause akathisia, although this condition is more common in people using conventional rather than atypical medication.

Akathisia can be effectively managed or prevented and the most effective treatment is the use of low-dose beta-adrenergic antagonists.

Anticholinergic medicines and benzodiazepines (see Chapter 9) are also effective in the treatment of akathisia. However, an atypical antipsychotic with a lower propensity to induce akathisia, such as olanzapine or quetiapine, may be a better alternative.

Pseudo-Parkinsonism

Symptoms of antipsychotic-induced Parkinsonism, or pseudo-Parkinsonism, include muscle stiffness, cogwheel rigidity, shuffling gait, stooped posture and drooling. Mask-like faces, abnormal slowness of movement (bradykinesia) and an indifference towards the environment (ataraxia), which are also part of the Parkinsonian syndrome, are often misdiagnosed as the negative symptoms of schizophrenia. Pseudo-Parkinsonism occurs in about 15 per cent of patients who are treated with an antipsychotic, usually developing within 5 to 90 days of starting treatment. Antipsychotic-induced Parkinsonism affects women twice as often as men, and the disorder can occur in all ages, although the elderly are particularly at risk. It is important to note that Parkinsonian side effects can be difficult to diagnose in some patients in practice because of the overlap of symptoms between this condition, negative symptoms and depressive symptoms. A failure to recognise and treat symptoms of Parkinsonism can lead to increased morbidity and mortality in patients. Anticholinergic medication can be used to treat symptoms of medicine-induced Parkinsonism, but it may be necessary to switch medication to an antipsychotic that has a low propensity for causing Parkinsonism. Most atypical antipsychotics cause fewer Parkinsonian side effects compared to conventional antipsychotics.

Case study

Pete is a 34-year-old man who has suffered from schizophrenia for six years and takes a flupenthixol decanoate depot injection to control his symptoms. Initially, he was happy to receive the injection from his care coordinator, but after about six months became increasingly unhappy about the injection, saying that it was turning him into a zombie and that his neck and muscles ached. At a review meeting, it was agreed that his flupenthixol depot should be tapered off in favour of risperidone (Risperdal Consta). After three months, Pete's mental state improved, he was hearing derogatory voices only on rare occasions and was more socially active. He was making frequent bus journeys to visit his grandmother who lived nearby.

It is clear that Pete was experiencing EPS as a result of taking flupenthixol. Flupenthixol decanoate is a conventional antipsychotic that blocks dopamine receptors in the therapeutic pathways, but also blocks dopamine in the nigrostriatal pathway, giving rise to EPS. Many patients who experience these types of side effects complain of muscle stiffness and painful muscles, particularly of the neck, jaws and limbs. After Pete's depot injection was switched to risperidone (which is an atypical), this caused fewer extrapyramidal symptoms through its blockade of serotonin as well as dopamine receptors (see page 143).

Tardive dyskinesia

Tardive dyskinesia is a delayed effect of antipsychotics and rarely occurs until after six months of treatment. The disorder consists of endless, complex abnormal involuntary, irregular (choreoathetoid) movements of the muscles of the head, limbs and trunk. Most common are darting, twisting and protruding movements of the tongue, chewing and lateral jaw movements, lip puckering and facial grimacing. Finger movements and hand-clenching are also common. The incidence has been estimated as from 32 per cent of patients after five years of conventional antipsychotic exposure to 68 per cent after 25 years of exposure (Glazer et al., 1993). In the elderly, tardive dyskinesia may develop in as many as 53 per cent of patients after three years of cumulative exposure to conventional antipsychotic usage. Women, those with diabetes, and patients with brain damage are at greatest risk of developing the condition (Woerner et al., 1998). It is important for you to remember that tardive dyskinesia can add to the subjective experience of disability and also to objective feelings of 'oddness', both of which affect rehabilitation and social inclusion. It is important to keep doses of antipsychotics low to minimise the risk of tardive dyskinesia in the first place, but also to minimise worsening of the condition once it has emerged. High-potency antipsychotics such as haloperidol should be avoided if possible in the high-risk groups. Consider a switch to low-potency or atypical antipsychotic medication with a low propensity for causing side effects.

Hormonal and sexual side effects

Earlier in the chapter, we explained that antipsychotics act in a non-therapeutic fourth dopamine pathway called the tuberoinfundibular pathway. Antipsychotic action of this system will result in hormonal or endocrinological side effects, including irregular periods and excessive discharge of breast milk (galactorrhoea) in women (Weiden et al., 1998) and excessive development of the breasts (gynaecomastia) and impotence in males due to **hyperprolactinaemia**. Identified risk factors for galactorrhoea are the use of conventional depot antipsychotic medications and long-term antipsychotic use. As previously mentioned, sexual side effects are common but are rarely reported by people with a psychosis.

All conventional antipsychotics have been associated with sexual dysfunction and the incidence of these side effects is underestimated. As many as 50 per cent of men taking antipsychotics experience impotence and ejaculatory problems. Impotence, decreased libido and changes in the quality of orgasm may be due to reduced testosterone or hyperprolactinaemia. Women may experience orgasmic dysfunction and reduced libido possibly due to alpha-adrenergic activity and calcium channel blockade.

Although sexual side effects can make conventional antipsychotic intolerable to many patients, clinicians often fail to ask about sexual dysfunction and patients tend not to report it to their professional carers spontaneously.

> ## Case study
>
> *Jack, a 25-year-old man, was admitted to hospital after he was found in the early hours of the morning in the street, muttering and shouting to himself. Part of his treatment plan included taking haloperidol 15mg per day in divided doses. After a week of haloperidol, he complained to his primary nurse that he was unhappy about his medication because it was making his genitals melt away, and he now feels that his genitals have changed to a woman's. He had not expressed this view before and the doctor was made aware of Jack's deteriorating condition. His medication was subsequently increased to 20mg per day. Jack repeated his claims that his genitals had melted due to the medication. Because of the high dose of haloperidol Jack was on, and also the nature of his complaint, the consultant psychiatrist ordered a prolactin levels test, which revealed that Jack had prolactin levels of 30mcg/L, which is way above the normal threshold. Haloperidol was tapered off in favour of quetiapine, which was titrated up. After a month of taking quetiapine, Jack no longer complained about his genitals melting away.*

Jack's case demonstrates the metaphorical way in which patients with psychosis can communicate. It also shows that it is important for you to recognise that conventional antipsychotics cause sexual side effects more often than not. Jack's mental state may be deteriorating, but in many cases patients with psychosis express themselves in metaphors (**secondary delusions**). When Jack said his medicine had made his genitals disappear, this was his attempt to explain the sexual side effects he was experiencing.

Non-extrapyramidal side effects of antipsychotics

In addition to blocking dopamine D_2 receptors in dopamine pathways, conventional antipsychotics in general also act on other receptors, such as the muscarinic, histamine and alpha-adrenergic receptors. This gives rise to different side effects because the way they act on non-dopamine receptors differs from medicine to medicine. This is a critical point to remember when choosing an antipsychotic. The following sections will describe the blockade of muscarinic, histamine and alpha-adrenergic receptors and how this causes side effects.

Muscarinic receptors

Muscarinic receptors are acetylcholine receptors found in the plasma membranes of some neurons and other cells. They play several roles, including acting as the main end-receptor stimulated by acetylcholine.

The blockade of muscarinic receptors causes adverse side effects such as dry mouth, blurred vision, constipation and cognitive blunting. In general, conventional antipsychotics that cause the most EPS are also known to exert a weak anticholinergic action. An example of such medicines is the butylphenones group, which includes haloperidol. Butylphenone blocks alpha-adrenergic receptors but has little or no action on the muscarinic receptors, thus causing few or no muscarinic side effects. By contrast, medicines that cause fewer EPS tend to cause pronounced cholinergic effects. The phenothiazines group of medicines is a good example of these types of medicines, which include chlorpromazine.

Alpha-adrenergic receptors

The adrenergic receptors are a class of receptors that are targets for the neurotransmitters noradrenaline and adrenaline. Many cells possess these receptors, and the excitatory binding of noradrenaline or adrenaline will generally cause the 'fight or flight' sympathetic response (see Chapter 4). There are two main groups of adrenergic receptors, alpha and beta, with several subtypes. We are concerned only with the actions of alpha receptors and a specific role of alpha$_1$ receptors involves smooth muscle contraction. They cause vasoconstriction in many blood vessels, including those of the skin, gastrointestinal system, kidney and brain. Blockade of these receptors causes dizziness, drowsiness and decreased blood pressure.

Histamine receptors

Histamine is a substance that plays a major role in many allergic reactions. It dilates blood vessels and makes the vessel walls abnormally permeable. Histamine receptors are proteins situated in various parts of the body that bind with histamine to produce a specific effect on the body. There are four known receptors, designated H_1 to H_4. Histamine H_1 is one of the most important receptors for modulating the internal clock, and is a main target for many medicines. When histamine reacts with these receptors, it alters the body's neurochemistry to make a person more awake and alert. The blockade of histamine receptors is associated with adverse side effects such as weight gain and drowsiness. In general, low-potency antipsychotics such as chlorpromazine and atypical antipsychotics such as olanzapine tend to block H_1, causing weight gain and metabolic syndrome, and this will be dealt with in later chapters. To test your understanding, please try Activity 7.7.

Activity 7.7   *Critical thinking*

- Why is olanzapine medication administered mostly before bedtime?

An outline answer is provided at the end of the chapter.

Haematological and hepatic effects

Antipsychotic side effects acting on the blood system include an increase or decrease in the number of white blood cells (leucocytosis or leucopenia), which usually occurs between six and eight weeks after antipsychotic initiation. This decrease in white blood cells is brought about by the suppressive effect some antipsychotics have on the bone marrow. In most cases, this condition is not permanent with the majority of antipsychotic medications, except for clozapine. A life-threatening blood condition is *agranulocytosis*, a condition where the granulocyte-producing ability of the bone marrow is severely diminished. This can occur with some conventional antipsychotic medication and it has a mortality rate as high as 30 per cent. This condition can occur within the first three months of antipsychotic treatment.

Antipsychotics have been linked to liver dysfunction; mild to moderate increases in transaminase (the enzyme promoting the addition to or the removal of oxygen from molecules) are normally detected early in the treatment phase and some patients experience liver dysfunction early during treatment with antipsychotics. *Cholestatic jaundice* is the yellowing of the skin caused by thickening of bile, obstruction of liver ducts, or generally by changes in liver cell function. Frequent blood monitoring is required in patients taking clozapine and this will be dealt with in more detail in later sections.

Allergic and dermatological effects

Allergic dermatitis occurs in a small percentage of patients, most commonly in those taking low-potency medicines. However, the most serious allergic adverse effects are **angioedema** and **exfoliative dermatitis**. Other antipsychotic adverse effects affecting the skin are photosensitivity and skin hyperpigmentation. *Hyperpigmentation* is a usually harmless condition in which patches of skin become darker in colour than the normal surrounding skin. *Photosensitivity* resembles severe sunburn and patients are usually warned to spend no more than 30 to 60 minutes in the sun and to use sunscreens. Skin hyperpigmentation occurs mainly with the chronic use of the medicine chlorpromazine and appears to bear a linear relationship with the dose.

Opthalmological effects

Thioridazine, one of the conventional antipsychotics, is linked to irreversible pigmentation of the retina when given in doses of more than 800mg a day. Chlorpromazine is associated with a relatively benign pigmentation of the eyes. Other ocular effects may range from inconvenient cornea changes to acute angle closure glaucoma, causing impairment of vision ranging from slight abnormalities to total blindness.

Neuroleptic malignant syndrome

Neuroleptic malignant syndrome (NMS) is a life-threatening, although rare, neurological disorder most often caused by an adverse reaction to antipsychotic medication. It generally presents with muscle rigidity, fever and delirium, and is associated with elevated **creatine phosphokinase**. NMS is a potentially fatal side effect of antipsychotic medication that can occur any time during the course of treatment. The motor and behavioural symptoms include muscular rigidity, dystonia, mutism and agitation. Other symptoms include excess salivation, elevated body temperature (hyperpyrexia), sweating and increased pulse and blood pressure. Laboratory findings include increased white blood count (WBC), liver enzymes, creatine phosphokinase, plasma myoglobin and myoglobinuria. The symptoms usually evolve over 72 hours, and the untreated symptoms can last for 10 to 14 days. The diagnosis is often missed during the early stages and withdrawal or agitation may mistakenly be considered to reflect increased psychosis. Men are affected more frequently than women and young patients are affected more commonly than older patients. The risk is also increased in agitated men who have received intramuscular injections of antipsychotic medication in high and rapidly escalating doses. The mortality rate can reach 30 per cent or higher when conventional antipsychotics are involved. The mechanism of how this serious condition arises is still not clear. Multiple factors probably contribute to NMS, including dehydration, comorbid medical conditions and agitation. Physical exhaustion, dehydration, **hyponatraemia**, young male gender, affective disorders, thyrotoxicosis, or prior brain pathology all increase the rate of this syndrome developing.

Weight gain

One of the commonest adverse side effects of treatment with dopamine receptor antagonists is weight gain. When chlorpromazine was introduced, most patients gained weight and similar problems have occurred to varying degrees with both conventional and atypical antipsychotics. As previously mentioned, excessive weight gain in a patient being treated with an antipsychotic renders them vulnerable to obesity-related illnesses such as cardiovascular diseases and non-insulin-dependent diabetes. The term *metabolic syndrome* has been used to describe this group of cardio-metabolic risk factors, and a recent meta-analysis (Newcomer, 2005) found that atypical antipsychotics such as olanzapine and clozapine were associated with a higher incidence of diabetes in patients. In contrast, risperidone and quetiapine were not associated with a higher incidence of developing diabetes. Clearly, metabolic syndrome presents a considerable health risk to patients and its prevention, or management once it has occurred, is very important.

Seizures

All antipsychotics reduce the seizure threshold to some degree, and therefore seizures are a potential early complication of antipsychotic treatment. The practical risk of seizures, however, is low, being 0.5–0.9 per cent of all patients taking antipsychotic treatment. Rapid increase of dosage (upward titration) is a risk factor and others include a history of seizures, CNS disease and EEG abnormalities.

In general, all antipsychotics exert similar types of side effects, but the extent to which each individual antipsychotic exerts particular effects varies from medicine to medicine. Table 7.1 shows the side-effects profile of different antipsychotics, with the severity varying from low to severe.

Name of drug	Orthostatic hypotension	Anticho-linergic effects	Sedation	Weight gain	EPS	Dose range (mg/day)
Chlorpromazine	+++	+++	++++	+++	++	200–800
Haloperidol	+	+	++	++	++++	1.5–30
Trifluperazine	+	+	++	+	++++	2–20
Clozapine	++	+	++++	++++	+	200–900
Sulpiride	++	++	+++	+++	+++	200–3200
Amisulpiride	+	+	++	+++	++	400–1200
Olanzapine	+	+	+++	++++	+/−	5–30
Risperidone	+	+/−	+++	+++	++	2–8
Quetiapine	+	+	++	+	+/−	50–800
Fluphenazine	+	+	+		+++	2.5–20
Pimozide	+	+	+	+	+++	1–10
Loxapine	++	+	++	++	++	10–100

Table 7.1: Side effects of commonly used antipsychotics
(Key: + = low risk, ++ = moderate risk, +++ = high risk, ++++ =severe risk)

Management of common antipsychotic side effects

As previously explained, the side effects of antipsychotics are many and varied, and some of these side effects are quite distressing. The key to successful treatment with antipsychotics largely depends on how patients tolerate these side effects or how well they are managed. The following list summarises the management of the most common side effects.

- **Tardive dyskinesia**: No effective treatment is known except discontinuation of the medicine or switching to an atypical antipsychotic such as clozapine. There is some evidence to suggest vitamin E has a protective effect against developing tardive dyskinesia.
- **Acute dystonia**: This can be treated by the administration of sublingual lorazepam or IM procyclidine. To prevent recurrence, prophylactic procyclidine should be given. A switch to second- or third-generation antipsychotics should be considered.
- **Acute akathisia**: Anticholinergic medicines are not very effective; diazepam, clonazepam and beta-blockers can be used as treatments. Alternatively, doses can be reduced or an alternative, probably low-potency, antipsychotic should be considered.
- **Acute pseudo-Parkinsonism**: Anticholinergic medication should be used or the dose should be reduced. Alternatively, medication can be switched to a second- or third-generation atypical antipsychotic such as olanzapine or aripiprazole.
- **Dry mouth, blurry vision, constipation**: Encourage fluid intake, particularly water, and a high-fibre diet and stool softeners for constipation. Use bethanecol for blurred vision.
- **Hypotension**: Ask the patient to dangle legs, and rise from bed or chair slowly. Decrease the dose of antipsychotic or give it in divided doses. Increase salt intake or use fludrocortisone.
- **Sexual side effects**: Reduce the antipsychotic dose or switch medication to a more appropriate one. Recommend treatment with cyproheptadine or bethanechol.

So far this chapter has dealt in detail with the mechanism of action of antipsychotics and how side effects are brought about. The willingness of people to take medication largely depends on how well they tolerate adverse side effects. The next case study summarises the clinical situations you are likely to meet in your daily practice.

Case study

Dave is a 26-year-old man admitted to an acute admission ward following a joint home visit by his care coordinator and a psychiatrist. On arrival, they noticed that Dave was having an argument with his mother. When Dave saw the two professionals enter the house, he went upstairs to his room and refused to see them. His mother reported that, for the past month, David had not been taking his prescribed medication (risperidone 6mg twice a day). She had observed his mental state deteriorating gradually, marked by periods of irritability and confrontational behaviour. He believed his neighbours had contracted a hit man to assassinate him. As a result, he rarely went out of the house and, when he did, it was only to the local market to buy fish, which he keeps in his room as he believes that the presence of fish will drive evil spirits continued . . .

away from the house. He was frequently heard muttering to himself, particularly at night. His appetite and sleep pattern were poor.

After much persuasion by his care coordinator, Dave eventually came downstairs and agreed to speak to her and the doctor. He confirmed the story about his neighbours and the fish, but was unwilling to take medication when the subject was brought up by the doctor. He believed the medication was poison and caused his jaws to ache. He agreed, however, to be admitted to hospital on a voluntary basis. As part of his treatment plan, his dosage of risperidone was increased to 10mg a day (4mg in the morning and 6mg at night). After three days in hospital, Dave's condition appeared to have deteriorated somewhat. He was more irritable and restless, and still complained of 'painful jaw' and of the medication being poison.

On a previous admission, Dave developed a good rapport with one of the nurses and it was during a discussion about his treatment that it transpired that Dave had stopped taking medication a few months after being discharged from hospital. He sees little point in taking medication once he is well. Also, the medicine made him restless and irritable and, in particular, he complained of inner tension and restlessness in his legs, which was only relieved by standing up and, even then, the relief was only temporary.

The nurse carried out an in-depth assessment of adverse side effects on Dave and it was apparent that Dave was experiencing a mild form of akathisia and dystonia. After documenting the finding in the patient's notes, the nurse informed the consultant doctor and, during a ward round, Dave's medication was reviewed. After much consultation with Dave, his medication was switched to olanzapine 10mg at night. Propranolol 20mg was also prescribed for two weeks. His primary nurse provided him with information about the medication and the possible side effects.

Gradually Dave experienced less restlessness and he began to take part in ward-based activities. His parents visited him regularly and were very pleased with the progress he was making. Initially, he was allowed to go home during the day and his mother reported that he kept himself busy, playing guitar and visiting friends. After 24 days as an inpatient, Dave was discharged back home on a maintenance dose of 7.5mg olanzapine. Dave was particularly concerned about gaining weight. He had a discussion with his primary care nurse about possible ways of keeping his weight under control. Of all the options discussed, he decided to resume regular swimming.

This case study is about a patient in the community who was non-adherent to medication. Not unusually, his family did not realise this, so it is important to look out for evidence of non-adherence. Once identified, it is possible to work with the patient in order to reduce the chances of relapse that may lead to hospitalisation. If Dave had told his care coordinator that he was not taking his medication because of adverse side effects, it would have been possible then to switch medication to one that Dave could tolerate better. It is likely that this would have resulted in Dave adhering better to his medication and therefore an admission to hospital could have been avoided. The key point for you here is the importance of a good rapport and honest communication with your patients. It is only when a patient is able to communicate freely with you that you are able to know exactly what is going on and this allows you to intervene appropriately.

Another contributory factor to Dave's suboptimal response to care is the relatively high dose of antipsychotic he was initially prescribed (risperidone 12mg daily). Risperidone doses of above

6mg tend to cause EPS and, clearly, Dave was suffering from symptoms consistent with akathisia. What is remarkable is that, due to poor recognition of akathisia, his risperidone dose was increased in the mistaken belief that his mental condition was deteriorating. Not surprisingly, this made his condition worse. This is not an uncommon scenario, particularly in a busy clinical setting where staff have limited time for a detailed assessment of a patient's needs. Unfortunately, poor assessment or limited attention to a patient's needs almost always leads to suboptimal care, thus denying the patient full benefits of treatment that he or she rightly deserves. Quite often in clinical practice, akathisia is mistaken for psychotic agitation and staff respond typically by increasing the antipsychotic dose, thereby exacerbating the problem, as in Dave's case. In this regard, you need to be fully conversant with side effects profiles of different antipsychotics. At times, it may not be possible to switch medication, as you will see in Activity 7.8.

Activity 7.8   *Critical thinking*

Look back at the last case study. Suppose it was not possible for Dave to switch medicines.

- What alternative care pathway would you have recommended to him?

An outline answer is provided at the end of the chapter.

Common treatment errors to avoid

The long-term use of antipsychotics, and atypical antipsychotics specifically, is associated with weight gain and cardiovascular disease. Patients should be screened for a familial history. Weigh the patient before they start antipsychotics to find out if they are already overweight or obese. A BMI of greater than 25 should indicate the person is overweight. If a patient gains more than 5 per cent of initial weight, discuss switching to another atypical antipsychotic.

Most antipsychotics can cause hypotension, so blood pressure should be checked before commencing antipsychotics and regularly for a few weeks afterwards. Also, patients can suffer hypotension after the administration of intramuscular short-acting low-potency antipsychotics. The patient should be advised to lie on his or her back (supine position) for 30 minutes after administration. Blood pressure should be taken before and after each intramuscular dose.

Akathisia is an extremely uncomfortable side effect, frequently misdiagnosed as psychotic agitation. It is important to routinely assess for the presence of akathisia, particularly in those prescribed high-potency antipsychotics. Patients taking antipsychotics and experiencing emotional blunting can be misconstrued as having negative symptoms. Anticholinergic medication should be used only to alleviate EPS; excessive use or abuse can cause a toxic psychosis. Monitor patients' fluid intake and be particularly vigilant for urinary retention in the elderly. Abrupt discontinuation of an antipsychotic is only advised in situations that have the potential to cause sudden death or severe adverse reaction. Patients should be advised that sudden withdrawal of medication can cause the discontinuation syndrome, which involves a number of symptoms including nausea, vomiting, diarrhoea, cold sweats and muscle aches and pains. Movement disorder (withdrawal dyskinesia) can appear within the first two to three weeks after discontinuation. Withdrawal dystonias, Parkinsonism and akathisia are known to occur within days of discontinuation.

What the patient needs to know

- You should explain to patients that most psychotic illness and schizophrenia are relapsing conditions and taking medication regularly is important to prevent relapse. Even if someone is fine, it is important to emphasise the importance of continual medication-taking to act as an insurance against relapse.
- It is important that you tell the patient the name of the medication, the dosage and the number of times the medicine is to be taken. You should emphasise the importance of taking medication with food or soon after mealtimes to avoid gastrointestinal irritation.
- Antipsychotic medications are not addictive, but coming off them should be done slowly to avoid unpleasant complications. The patient should discuss this with the prescriber if he or she wishes to stop taking the antipsychotics.
- You should explain in simple terms, depending on the level of the patient's understanding, the likely side effects the patient may suffer. In particular, you should explain EPS such as akathisia, tardive dyskinesia, dystonia and Parkinsonism for those prescribed conventional antipsychotics.
- Patients in their first episode of illness should be informed that treatment is likely to be for a year, but treatment for those who have had two or more episodes is likely to be indefinite, as stated by the National Institute for Health and Clinical Excellence (NICE) guidelines.
- You should explain to the patient the role of psychostimulants such as cocaine, amphetamine and cannabis in triggering or worsening psychosis.
- If medication to relieve EPS is prescribed, it should be continued for a few weeks after antipsychotics have been discontinued.
- The patient should be warned that, because most antipsychotics can cause cardiac arrhythmia, they can be fatal if taken in overdose.
- Most antipsychotics can cause drowsiness due to their effect on histamine receptors; you should warn the patient not to drive a car or operate machinery while taking antipsychotic medication.

Chapter summary

Schizophrenia is the most common of all psychotic disorders and perhaps the most widely investigated. It affects 0.1 per cent of the population. The commonest types of symptoms for schizophrenia are hallucinations, delusions, thought disorder, bizarre behaviour, negative cognitive deficits, and affective symptoms.

Some medicines and many physical illnesses can cause psychotic symptoms. Positive symptoms of psychosis are due to an increase in dopamine activity in the synapse in the mesolimbic region of the brain. This is corrected by blocking post-synaptic dopamine receptors with antipsychotics. Apart from blocking post-synaptic receptors, dopamine also blocks other regions and receptors in the brain, giving rise to adverse side effects. The older conventional antipsychotics cause more EPS by blocking dopamine receptors in the

continued . . .

nigrostriatal pathway. Newer, atypical antipsychotics have a better, more tolerable, side-effects profile than conventional forms, but they still have worrying side effects such as sedation and weight gain. Antipsychotic medications are generally started at low doses and titrated up in an effort to minimise side effects. The multiple receptor binding profile of atypical antipsychotics has been linked to these medicines causing cardio-metabolic problems. Clozapine is effective for people who have responded poorly to other antipsychotics. Blood should be taken regularly to monitor for neutropaenia. The medicines to prescribe should be driven by the patient's preference and lifestyle.

Activities: brief outline answers

Activity 7.1 Electrolytes test (page 138)

Electrolytes imbalance will generally cause toxic confusional states, particularly in the elderly.

Activity 7.2 Thyroid function (page 138)

You should recommend a thyroid function test. She is restless and thought disordered, which are common signs of psychosis due to excess thyroxin. Thyrotoxicosis is a genetically inheritable disease.

Activity 7.3 Urine sample (page 138)

You should screen the urine for illicit medicines.

Activity 7.4 Haloperidol (page 143)

Haloperidol will make negative symptoms worse. To improve the situation, suggest an alternative such as an atypical antipsychotic.

Activity 7.5 Sexual dysfunction (page 144)

Out of the three, the medication you would expect to cause sexual dysfunction is haloperidol.

Activity 7.6 Trifluperazine (page 145)

Dave is most likely experiencing akathisia: he is young, taking conventional antipsychotic and his restlessness coincided with initiation of trifluperazine. In this case, a change of antipsychotic is the best course of action. If this is not possible, Dave can be given beta-blockers or benzodiazepines.

Activity 7.7 Olanzapine (page 149)

Apart from its antipsychotic effect due to its blockade of D_2 receptors, olanzapine blocks histamine and alpha-adrenergic receptors, giving rise to drowsiness. If given at night, it can have a dual role of relieving psychotic symptoms and helping a person to sleep. By contrast, if olanzapine is given during daytime, its sedative effects can interfere with normal social functioning.

Activity 7.8 Alternative to risperidone (page 154)

The dosage of risperidone could be decreased and concomitant beta-blocker medicines or lorazepam could be prescribed to alleviate symptoms of akathisia.

Further reading

Stahl, SM (2008) *Stahl's Essential Psychopharmacology: Neuroscientific basis and practical application*, 3rd edition. Cambridge: Cambridge University Press.

Stahl, SM (2009) *Stahl's Essential Psychopharmacology: The prescriber's guide*, 3rd edition. Cambridge: Cambridge University Press.

These are very good books that explain psychotropic medicines well, with good illustrations.

Taylor, D, Paton, C and Kerwin, R (2007) *The Maudsley Prescribing Guidelines*, 9th edition. London: Informa Healthcare.

This is a very useful, easy-to-understand, evidence-based prescribing and general medicines management manual.

Useful websites

www.bnf.org

The *British National Formulary* is very useful for finding out about drug information, including normal dosages, interactions and side effects.

www.medicines.org.uk/emc

This website supplies very detailed information on medicine side effects and interactions.

www.rethink.org

This very useful website publishes material on service users and carers of people with serious mental illness.

Chapter 8
Management and treatment of dementias

Chapter aims

By the end of this chapter, you should be able to:

*   outline the main clinical features of dementia;
*   describe anti-dementia medication and its mechanism of action;
*   recognise the side effects of anti-dementia medicines;
*   describe common mistakes to avoid in the treatment of dementia;
*   communicate necessary information to patients and carers.

Introduction

Case study

Marjorie is 68 years old and retired from her job as a personal secretary after 35 years. She has noticed that driving long distances confuses her; she frequently forgets how to get to her destination, and because of this she has stopped driving altogether. Her troubles with memory have deteriorated so much that coping with the activities of daily living has been getting progressively more difficult. Over the past months, her short-term memory has deteriorated and she has suffered gastrointestinal problems that led to a dramatic weight loss, causing her to become depressed. Recently, she was rushed to hospital after she found it difficult to walk or talk; she was weak and unable to absorb food properly.

After several investigations, doctors could not find the cause of Marjorie's gastrointestinal problems, but took a particular interest in the results of CT scan. This and her non-existent short-term memory led her doctor to conclude that Marjorie was suffering from Alzheimer's disease. However, her long-term memory was still intact. Because of her deteriorating physical and mental health, her only daughter moved in to look after her full time. Her daughter was able to slow down Marjorie's deterioration by monitoring what she ate and how often. Her daughter's good care was essential for her survival. However, Marjorie's condition gradually deteriorated further, which had a hugely stressful effect on her daughter. Because of this, Marjorie was admitted to a nursing home where her daughter regularly visits her.

Dementia is a progressive and largely irreversible mental health condition that is characterised by a widespread impairment of mental function. Although dementia is far more common in the older population, it may occur at any stage of adulthood. It is a non-specific illness in which areas of cognition, memory, attention, language or problem-solving are affected. For dementia to be diagnosed, symptoms normally should be present for at least six months, but if cognitive dysfunction has been seen for only a short time, especially less than a week, it must be termed delirium.

This chapter will first briefly review the mechanisms underlying Alzheimer's disease and describe the common clinical features of the condition, before discussing the treatment and care of people with dementia. The final section of the chapter covers treatment errors to avoid and what you as a nurse need to discuss with patients who have dementia and their carers.

Alzheimer's disease and amyloid cascade theory

Dementia and Alzheimer's disease

In 1907, Alois Alzheimer first described the illness that later assumed his name. According to experts, without the introduction of disease-modifying treatments, Alzheimer's disease is poised to increase rapidly throughout the world; current estimates are that it will quadruple over the next 40 years to affect one in every 85 people. Although the cause of Alzheimer's disease is not clearly understood, it is thought that genetic factors play an important part. Approximately 40 per cent of people with this condition have a family history of dementia. Also, the concordance rate for illness in monozygotic (identical) twins is high: 43 per cent compared to that of dizygotic twins, which is 8 per cent. The risk factors of developing Alzheimer's dementia include being female, having a first-degree relative who has the disorder, and having a history of head injury. The brain of someone with Alzheimer's is characterised by shrinkage (atrophy) and enlarged cerebral ventricles. It is thought that the neurotransmitters acetylcholine and noradrenaline are under-active in those with Alzheimer's disease. Cholinergic antagonists, such as atropine, impair cognitive abilities, whereas cholinergic agonists, such as physostigmine, enhance them.

The cognitive functions that are affected in dementia include general intelligence, learning, memory, language, problem-solving, orientation, perception, attention, concentration, judgement and social ability. A person's personality may also be affected. The illness is mostly progressive and permanent, but if there is an underlying cause that can be treated, the condition may be reversible. Approximately 15 per cent of the people with dementia have reversible illness if treatment begins before irreversible damage takes place.

Amyloid cascade theory

This theory originated from early findings of profound acetylcholine neural loss in people with Alzheimer's dementia. The death of these acetylcholine neurons is brought about by *amyloid plaques*. Amyloids are an aggregation of low molecular weight protein that forms plaques outside neurons. These plaques interfere with the normal biochemical function of the neurons and cause conditions such as inflammation of the neuron, and release of toxic chemicals including cytokines and free radicals. Further, these amyloid plaques induce the conversion of cell microtubules into tangles, which will lead to neuronal cell dysfunction that ultimately leads to neuronal cell death. Genetic studies have confirmed the amyloid cascade theory.

Clinical features of dementia

Case study

David is a 58-year-old man who has worked as a painter and decorator for most of his life. He is married with three grown-up children and five grandchildren. Recently, his wife noticed that David was doing 'silly things' without realising it. On a number of occasions, he had been paid cash for his work and, when his wife asked him about the money, he would have no idea what she was talking about. Sometimes David would leave the money in the car or lose it completely. He would often get irritable for no reason. Lately, he has had problems remembering the names of his children. It was at this point that David saw his GP and was referred to a specialist who diagnosed Alzheimer's disease.

The onset of dementia is insidious, and symptoms manifest themselves slowly over a period of years. At the initial stages, patients show fatigue, difficulty in sustaining mental performance and a tendency to fail when a task is new, complex or requires a shift in problem-solving strategy. One of the early, prominent and classical signs in people with dementia is memory impairment, especially those with dementia of Alzheimer's type. The case of David's forgetfulness is typical of someone showing early signs of Alzheimer's disease. The ability to perform activities of daily living, such as shopping, managing finances and using the telephone, is lost earlier in the course of the illness, while abilities such as eating and grooming are lost at later stages. Patients in residential care with dementia can forget how to get back to their rooms after going to the toilet. Also, those with Alzheimer's and vascular dementia can suffer abilities in language processing and this can be characterised by vague, imprecise or **circumstantial speech**. They may have difficulties in naming objects, and may undergo personality changes that can be profoundly disturbing for the patient's family. The patient may become quite introverted and unconcerned about their relatives, or they may become very hostile to them. Patients with frontal and temporal lobe dementia may experience marked changes in their personality that include being explosive and irritable. It is estimated that up to 30 per cent of patients with dementia (Alzheimer's type) have hallucinations and up to 40 per cent have paranoid delusions and are generally hostile to the family. In the end, people with dementia will need supervision and assistance with the basic tasks of daily living, which may be particularly distressing. Therefore, you need to identify the activities of daily living that are important to the patient and his or her family so that treatment and management can be tailored to target these activities. More importantly, in collaboration with the patient and carers, you should periodically revisit the issue of which activities are most important, as priorities may change over the course of treatment. People with dementia face a gradual but downward progression of disease symptoms, with an average timescale from onset of illness to death of between eight and ten years.

Care and management of people with dementia

Many of the effective treatments for dementia are centred on boosting the availability of the neurotransmitter acetylcholine in the brain synapses. Acetylcholine is broken down by two enzymes – acetylcholinesterase and butylcholinesterase – into the inactive compounds choline and acetate. Inhibiting (disabling) these enzymes will result in the accumulation of acetylcholine in the cholinergic system, rendering more acetylcholine available for neurotransmission. Increased levels of acetylcholine in the cholinergic system improve memory and cognitive ability. It therefore follows that substances that block (antagonise) acetylcholine receptors in normal humans produce memory disturbances similar to those seen in Alzheimer's. An example of such a substance is scolopamine. Overall, it is important for you to tailor your nursing intervention around the recovery approach.

At first glance it may be thought that the current emphasis on promoting 'recovery' has little relevance to people with dementia. However, there are striking similarities between the values and aspirations of the recovery model and the principles of person-centred care that guide dementia care in the NHS. In this regard, you aim to promote people's capacity to care for themselves for as a long as they are able to do so. One way you can achieve this is by combining pharmacological with non-pharmacological approaches, which is what we will look at next.

Non-pharmacological approaches to care of people with dementia

There is compelling evidence that the care of people with dementia, especially towards the end of their lives, is less than optimal (Ballard et al., 2001). Retrospective case-note studies demonstrate inadequate care in both psychiatric and acute hospital wards (Sampson et al., 2006). Life expectancy is more emphatically curtailed by dementia than it is by other mental health syndromes, yet the evidence for suboptimal care persists, especially in the later stages of the illness. In a retrospective survey of carers in England, McCarthy et al. (1997) reported a host of common signs and symptoms experienced by people with dementia in the last year of life: confusion, urinary incontinence, pain, low mood, constipation and loss of appetite. The study found similar frequencies of such symptoms in cancer patients, but people with dementia experienced the symptoms for longer.

The physical health of people with advanced dementia needs increasing consideration as the condition progresses and there are specific symptoms and signs associated with dying. Of particular note is that people with dementia tend to have difficulties with nutritional intake and these can be present even during the early stages of the illness. The impact of poor nutrition is profound and this may be due to an inability to request food or drinks, feed themselves or recognise food, or due to refusing to eat or having significant problems with swallowing food. While it is difficult to reverse the problem of malnutrition in people with late-stage dementia, you should nonetheless treat malnutrition in order to maintain or to slow down deterioration that may be due to poor nutrition. You should bear in mind that older people with dementia generally have a lower BMI and this is usually associated with higher frequency and severity of behavioural problems.

Bladder and bowel function are compromised, and incontinence of urine is common, which itself can threaten skin integrity, causing discomfort. You should seek advice from a continence specialist as this can often be helpful. Constipation, which can sometimes lead to impaction or overflow incontinence, can occur when the diet or fluid intake is poor, or when medication slows bowel transit times. Immobility and reduced awareness of the call to stool make matters worse. Constipation itself impedes bladder function and discomfort, pain or toxicity can follow. The person may become more confused or more agitated. A common sign of constipation is the tendency to lean to the side. Therefore you should be incorporate strategies that reduce the risk of constipation, such as adequate fluid intake, encouraging a high-fibre diet and promoting exercise.

General levels of functioning need attention, and the right amount of support should be provided to allow as much independence as possible while still maintaining the person's dignity. In addition to physical care, non-pharmacological care of people with Alzheimer's does include techniques that help compensate for cognitive losses. For example, you can employ the use of memory books, which contain important pieces of information that may be forgotten by the affected patient, as well as environmental modifications (for example, improvements in lighting and establishment of a quiet environment) that promote intellectual functioning. You should individualise the non-pharmacological care of people with Alzheimer's disease according to the stage of deterioration the patient is at. You should pay particular attention to the patient's safety, even in the early stages, and the use of technology can be particularly useful, as illustrated by the next case study.

Case study

Peter is a 76-year-old man who was diagnosed with Alzheimer's dementia soon after his wife died a year ago. It was reported on a number of occasions that Peter was found outside during the day in his pyjamas, appearing disorientated and in need of reassurance. His only daughter, who lives about 80 miles away, was visiting him frequently but was finding it difficult and therefore was becoming distressed. Because of the safety risk Peter presented, an electronic device with a recording of his daughter's voice was installed at his front door. This voice device was activated every time he approached the front door, telling him not to go out and wait for homecare staff to arrive. There were no reports of Peter wandering outside the house distressed after the device was installed. His daughter reported reduced levels of stress and distress.

We can see from the case study how the use of technology can be usefully employed to assist people with dementia. Helpful equipment is available that may support the independence of people with dementia (see 'Useful websites' at the end of the chapter). Assistive technology can not only enable people with dementia to live more independently, it may also help to support and reassure their carers. As much as assistive care is helpful, it is not the answer for every patient with dementia. In the main, it can be useful to those patients who are still in the early stages of the illness. Patients at this stage of disease may also benefit from being discouraged from performing certain activities of daily living in which they have shown impairment (for example, lighting the gas cooker or using a telephone).

However, as patients progressively deteriorate to the later stages of Alzheimer's disease, deficits in cognition and functioning become more profound. At this stage, it may be appropriate to introduce non-pharmacological interventions to focus on behavioural disturbances. Before you proceed further, you need to try Activity 8.1.

Activity 8.1   *Critical thinking*

Good physical healthcare is very important in people with dementia.

• What are the key physical healthcare interventions required to optimise patient well-being?

An outline answer is provided at the end of the chapter.

Pharmacological approaches to dementia

Cholinesterase inhibitors have a useful place in arresting the rate of memory and cognitive decline in patients. The only cholinesterase inhibitors approved for the treatment of Alzheimer's disease are donepezil, rivastigmine and galantamine. The NMDA receptor antagonist memantine is the only non-cholinesterase inhibitor approved for the treatment of Alzheimer's disease.

Cholinesterase inhibitors

Randomised, placebo-controlled clinical trials of cholinesterase inhibitors have included patients with mainly mild to moderate Alzheimer's disease and have shown significant benefits with respect to cognition, daily function and behaviour. The condition of patients who are taking these medicines can remain stable for a year or more and then it may decline, though at a rate that is slower than that of untreated patients. In other words, although these medicines may not be able to arrest intellectual decline in patients, they are able to slow down the rate at which deterioration takes place.

The European Federation of Neurological Societies has published recommendations for the diagnosis and management of Alzheimer's disease. On the basis of available research evidence, treatment with cholinesterase inhibitors is recommended even for mild or early disease; no specific cholinesterase inhibitor is recommended over another. In 2006, the American Association for Geriatric Psychiatry published practice recommendations that also emphasise treatment with approved medications for cognitive symptoms, as well as symptomatic treatment for neuro-psychiatric manifestations, such as depression and psychosis, and issues related to safety, such as driving, living alone and medication administration. In the UK, NICE guidelines (2009a) recommend that the three acetylcholinesterase inhibitors, donepezil, galantamine and rivastigmine, are options in the management of patients with Alzheimer's disease of moderate severity only. Before you proceed to the next section, you need to try Activity 8.2.

Activity 8.2   *Critical thinking*

Albert is a 72-year-old man with Alzheimer's, who is known to have enjoyed music and dancing in his youth. He is currently quite restless and agitated for no obvious reason.

• How might you get Albert to be settled and less agitated?

An outline answer is provided at the end of the chapter.

All currently available cholinesterase inhibitors (donezepil, rivastigmine and galantamine) show some evidence of a beneficial effect on patients with respect to activities of daily living. *Donepezil* is mainly used to increase levels of acetylcholine in the cortical region of the brain and therefore improve a patient's cognition. Furthermore, donepezil should improve a patient's behavioural disturbances, such as apathy, depression, anxiety and disinhibition. It is recommended as a treatment option for people with moderate to severe Alzheimer's disease only, and it has no effect on people suffering from vascular dementia. It can take up to six weeks before any improvements in the patient's memory can be noticed. In many cases, it can take several months before the degenerative process of Alzheimer's disease can be arrested. The NICE guideline (2009a) recommends that only specialists in dementia should prescribe and review these medicines. A review of the patient's treatment should be carried out every six months. Also, the views of the carer should always be sought at any given time. The normal doses for this medicine are 5mg once a day and this can be increased to 10mg a day.

Galantamine has been used for decades in Eastern Europe and the Soviet Union for various indications, such as the treatment of sensory and motor dysfunction associated with disorders of the CNS. It is a selective, competitive and reversible inhibitor of acetylcholine esterase and is suitable for the symptomatic treatment of people with mild to moderately severe Alzheimer's disease. It has been found to be effective in vascular dementia as well. In addition, galantamine enhances the action of acetylcholine on nicotinic receptors, thereby improving cognition in people with dementia. The maintenance dosage is 16–24mg daily.

Rivastigmine is an acetylcholinesterase and butyrylcholinesterase inhibitor, licensed in the UK. It was developed by Marta Weinstock-Rosin in Israel, and is useful in the symptomatic treatment of people with mild to moderately severe Alzheimer's dementia. Rivastigmine has been shown to provide meaningful symptomatic effects that may allow patients to remain independent and 'be themselves' for longer. In particular, rivastigmine appears to show marked positive treatment effects in patients showing a more aggressive form of Alzheimer's disease, such as those with a younger age of onset or a poor nutritional status, or those experiencing symptoms such as delusions or hallucinations (Gauthier et al., 2006). For example, the presence of hallucinations appears to be a predictor of especially strong responses to rivastigmine, both in Alzheimer's and other illnesses such as Parkinson's disease (Touchon et al., 2006). These effects might reflect the additional inhibition of butyrylcholinesterase, which is implicated in symptom progression and might provide added benefits over medicines that selectively inhibit acetylcholinesterase (Gauthier et al., 2006). The usual maintenance dosage is 3–6mg twice daily taken with food to minimise incidences of nausea.

All cholinesterase inhibitors cause similar side effects; the most common are nausea, vomiting, appetite loss, increased gastric acid secretion, weight loss, insomnia and dizziness. These side effects tend to occur early during the treatment process and most are transient. For general side effects management, see the sections on the management of specific side effects with mood stabilisers (Chapter 6), antipsychotics (Chapter 7) and antidepressants (Chapter 5). You should note that this medicine can exacerbate asthma or other pulmonary disease. Donepezil can be lethal in overdose and can cause a cholinergic crisis, which is characterised by nausea, vomiting, salivation, sweating, bradycardia and hypotension, followed by increased muscle weakness, respiratory depression and convulsions. If you suspect that someone has taken an overdose of donezepil, you should notify the doctor without delay. The most likely treatment for donepezil is atropine 1–2mg intravenously and this can be increased depending on the condition of the patient.

Non-cholinesterase inhibitor memantime

Memantine is an N-methyl-D-aspartate (NMDA) receptor antagonist that blocks the effects of unusually elevated levels of glutamate that may lead to neuronal dysfunction. It is used in the treatment of people with moderate to severe dementia. Clinical trials have also shown memantine to be effective in targeting functional decline associated with vascular dementia. For example, a 28-week, double-blind study involving patients with moderate to severe Alzheimer's disease found that patients receiving memantine 20mg/day experienced substantially slower functional deterioration than patients treated with a placebo, as measured by changes in activities of daily living (Wilcock et al., 2002). The recommended maintenance dosage is 10mg twice daily. Combination therapy with memantine has also been found to yield a functional benefit for patients with Alzheimer's disease. In a 24-week, double-blind trial involving patients already receiving donepezil for moderate to severe Alzheimer's disease, patients who had memantine 20mg/day added to their existing donepezil regimen experienced a significantly smaller decrease in the ability to perform activities of daily living (van Dyck et al., 2006). More significantly, a Cochrane systematic review has concluded that memantine has a beneficial effect on CNS activity and is a potential treatment for Alzheimer's disease, and for vascular and mixed dementia. It also has a beneficial effect on cognitive function in patients with moderate to severe Alzheimer's disease and those with vascular dementia. More notably, its adverse effects profile and tolerability are good and agitation is less common with memantine. However, its effect on people with mild to moderate Alzheimer's disease is unclear (Areosa et al., 2005).

Unfortunately, behavioural and psychiatric symptoms typically increase with disease progression in people with Alzheimer's disease. The most commonly experienced symptoms tend to be anxiety, depression and psychotic symptoms. As such, you need to take account of the presence of these symptoms in your care of people with Alzheimer's disease and it is this we will look at next.

Management of the psychiatric symptoms of dementia

Not surprisingly, available evidence suggests that depression is very common in people with Alzheimer's disease. At least 25 per cent of patients are likely to experience depression at the time of, or just before, the onset of the illness. In patients for whom medication is considered appropriate, SSRIs are commonly used, but TCAs are generally avoided, since their anticholinergic effects can cause or exacerbate confusion. Also, their cardiotoxic profile renders them unsuitable for use in the elderly. Please try Activity 8.3 before continuing.

Activity 8.3   *Critical thinking*

Jan is an 86-year-old lady with Alzheimer's dementia. You notice that her dietary intake has been poor lately and she is rather restless. Also, you notice that her stomach is slightly distended and that she has been refusing to take medication lately.

- How might you encourage her to take medication and food?

An outline answer is provided at the end of the chapter.

Delusions and hallucinations may sometimes occur in people with early Alzheimer's disease, but the occurrence of agitation, delusions, hallucinations and irritability early in the course of illness also raises the possibility of an alternative diagnosis, such as dementia with Lewy bodies (DLB) (Kaplan and Saddock, 1998). In any event, treatment with antipsychotic medication may be helpful, but these medicines should be used with extreme caution because of their tendency to cause adverse effects in the elderly in a profound way. If antipsychotics are to be administered, you need to manage side effects aggressively should they occur. For the management of antipsychotic-induced side effects, you need to refer to Chapter 7. The next section deals with the importance of providing support to caregivers but, before you move to this section, please try Activity 8.4.

Activity 8.4   *Decision-making*

Ahmed, a third-year student nurse, was on practice learning experience in a nursing home. One day, at lunchtime, he noticed Jeff, a resident, using his hands instead of cutlery to eat with. Ahmed rightly thought Jeff was having problems using cutlery, so he assisted him with his meal. However, he was stopped from assisting Jeff by the staff nurse, who insisted that 'Jeff is doing all right'.

- Do you agree with the staff nurse's view? If so, why?

An outline answer is provided at the end of the chapter.

Caregiver support

The Alzheimer's Society estimates that there are about 600,000 people in the UK acting as primary carers for people with dementia (**www.alzheimers.org.uk**). Evidence suggests that carers of people with dementia experience greater stress than carers of other older people (Moise et al., 2004). This comes as no surprise, as it can be a physically and emotionally draining experience that can bring irreversible changes to people's lives and relationships. Depression, emotional and physical exhaustion, and general poor health are common in carers. Many carers of people with dementia are old themselves, with physical frailty and health conditions of their own. You should routinely offer support, assistance with day-to-day caring and access to respite and short breaks, support groups, online groups and assistance with financial benefits, such as the carer's allowance.

Common treatment errors to avoid

Prior to commencing medication, you should ensure that the patient has undergone a full physical check-up that may include full blood count, liver function test, electrolytes and kidney function. Ensure that medication is taken with food to avoid gastrointestinal irritation. Good fluid intake is also very important and should be encouraged. If possible, the use of TCAs should be avoided in the elderly because of their tendency to cause drowsiness and constipation. If they are to be prescribed, they should be administered at night to minimise the incidence of daytime sedation. If antipsychotics are prescribed, you should be particularly vigilant for the occurrence of adverse side effects. The elderly are particularly sensitive to the disabling effects of EPS – Chapter 7.

What the patient and carers need to know

- Alzheimer's dementia is a progressively deteriorating illness that affects a person's memory and cognitive abilities.
- There is currently no cure for Alzheimer's disease and other related dementias, but there are some treatments that can temporarily help with some of the symptoms.
- It is common for people with dementia to have poor dietary intake, therefore patients should be encouraged to eat more and to follow a good diet to help with general well-being.
- Poor physical health is very common in people suffering from dementia. Patients may be taking medication for physical health conditions in addition to medicines to relieve symptoms of dementia. Check for possible medicines interactions and inform relatives where appropriate.

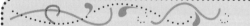

Chapter summary

Dementia is a condition that is characterised by gradual memory and cognitive impairment, mostly in elderly people. There are many forms of dementia but the most common is Alzheimer's disease and the prevalence of this illness is set to increase fourfold in the next 40 years. Alzheimer's disease is thought to be caused by a reduction in acetylcholine in the brain. Therefore, the treatment of Alzheimer's disease symptoms aims to correct acetylcholine deficiency and this is achieved by using cholinesterase inhibitors. Donezepil, galantamine and rivastigmine are the main cholinesterase inhibitors used in the treatment of Alzheimer's disease. In addition to patients suffering symptoms of dementia, they may also experience depression and other mental health problems. Therefore, it is important for you to be vigilant for the presence of these problems. You should also use non-pharmacological approaches to supplement the use of medicines and involve carers in the treatment of people with dementia.

Activities: brief outline answers

Activity 8.1 Physical healthcare interventions (page 164)

You should ensure a good diet and sufficient fluid intake, adequate sleep, adequate exercise during the day that involves adequate mental stimulation, and good oral hygiene. Always promote good bowel movements (e.g. through a high-fibre diet, fluids, exercise) to limit the chances of constipation.

Activity 8.2 Albert's restlessness (page 165)

Quite possibly, Albert is bored and the use of multidimensional activities can be very useful in this situation. He is known to be interested in music, so activities along these lines might be helpful.

Activity 8.3 Constipation (page 167)

It is important to assess whether Jan is constipated or not. Constipation is relatively common in the elderly. Jan has a distended stomach, restlessness and poor appetite. All these can be signs of constipation. Initially, you should promote good bowel movements by encouraging exercise, a high-fibre diet and drinking plenty of fluids.

Activity 8.4 Encouraging independence (page 167)

The staff nurse is correct. It is important for dementia patients to retain independence as much as possible. Although Jeff has lost the skill to use cutlery, at least he has not lost the skill to feed himself using his hands without assistance. The aim is to promote independence as much as possible.

Further reading

Martin, G and Sabbagh, M (2010) *Palliative Care for Advanced Alzheimer's and Dementia: Guidelines and standards for evidence-based care.* New York: Springer.

This is a very good book that offers practical advice for those looking after people with advanced dementia.

Mittelman, M (2003) *Counseling the Alzheimer's Care Giver: A resource for health care professionals.* Chicago, IL: American Medical Association Press.

This book is useful for those who intend to give carers support, advice and information.

Useful websites

www.alzheimers.org.uk

This is a very useful site that provides information about dementia in general and Alzheimer's disease in particular, including care and treatment and current research breakthroughs.

www.atdementia.org.uk

This website brings together information about assistive technology, which has the potential to support the independence and leisure opportunities of people with dementia.

www.carersuk.org

This website provides a forum for carers in the UK. Carers have the opportunity to voice and share their experiences to other carers and professionals alike.

Chapter 9
Management and treatment
of anxiety disorders

Introduction

Case study

Just before she sat her A-level exams, Amy experienced a state of uneasiness and worry because of her fear of failing. After the exams, however, she continued to worry, even about things she considered minor, and was unable to stop herself from worrying. In addition to worry and fear, she experienced somatic symptoms such as poor concentration and poor appetite. Her experiences impacted on her studies in several ways. She felt consistently in a state of anxiety, and at times would have panic attacks. She found it difficult to leave her house, as she was worried about having a panic attack on the journey to school. In addition, Amy encountered difficulties with classes and concentration on her work. She felt too embarrassed to tell her teachers about the problem and, as a result, she did not do well in her exams. Much later, she sought help from her GP and was diagnosed with anxiety and referred for counselling.

In common parlance, 'anxiety' is an unpleasant state of mental uneasiness or concern about some uncertain event, or a state of restlessness and agitation. Anxiety may be accompanied by a distressing sense of oppression or tightness in the stomach. Anxiety disorders probably existed long before recorded history (Anderson, 2007) and are not unique to human beings, although human anxiety appears to be the most complex. The earliest interpretations of anxiety disorders appear to be mostly spiritual; early spiritual treatments of the disorder somewhat resemble modern psychotherapies. It is also interesting that ancient and traditional natural remedies for anxiety have some surprising similarities to modern medicines.

Anxiety and anxiety disorders have played substantial roles in human history, most prominently in times of hardship, war or social change. In more pleasant times, however, societies tend to embrace the illusion that anxiety is a minor issue that deserves little attention or respect and it is easily ignored. Lack of interest in the fundamental nature of anxiety has often left societies ill-prepared for unforeseen challenges.

Anxiety is a normal emotion under threatening circumstances and is thought to be part of the evolutionary 'fight or flight' reaction to aid survival. Not only is it normal to be anxious, it is also adaptive. Normally, a balance exists between the mechanisms that produce neural excitation and inhibition and, in such cases, anxiety levels remain within normal limits. Should this balance be lost, anxiety becomes problematic and psychiatric symptoms develop. This chapter will initially provide an overview of anxiety symptoms and how they arise before discussing in more depth the medicines used to treat anxiety and their management. In the final sections, common treatment errors and what patients and carers need to know are covered.

Symptoms of anxiety

The idea of anxiety as a psychiatric disorder is evolving rapidly. Anxiety is characterised by core symptoms of excessive fear and worry. This is in contrast to depression where the core symptoms are depressed mood, and loss of interest and pleasure. Anxiety symptoms overlap considerably with those of major depression (see Chapter 5 on depression), in particular sleep disturbance, concentration difficulties, fatigue and **psychomotor arousal**. There are different types of anxiety disorder and they all have a great deal of symptom overlap with each other (see below). Also, people tend to have anxiety disorders when they have other psychiatric disorders, such as depression, schizophrenia, substance misuse and bipolar disorders.

In general, patients with anxiety experience some of the following symptoms: trembling, feeling shaky, restlessness, muscle tension, shortness of breath, smothering sensation, rapid heartbeat (tachycardia), sweating and cold hands and feet, light-headedness, dizziness, tingling of the skin, frequent urination, diarrhoea, feelings of unreality, difficulty in falling asleep, impaired attention and concentration, and nervousness. Some of these symptoms are present in one type of anxiety but may not be present in another – a complex situation that we will turn to now.

Overlapping symptoms of different types of anxiety disorder

Anxiety disorders encompass a broad group of psychiatric problems and, like depression, have many underlying causes (Preston et al., 2008). Some appear to be clearly related to biochemical abnormalities, while others seem to have a mainly psychological or emotional origin. There are at least five different types of anxiety disorder:

- generalised anxiety disorder (GAD);
- phobias;
- panic disorders;
- obsessive compulsive anxiety disorders;
- trauma associated anxiety disorders;
- social anxiety/phobia.

All types of anxiety disorder have the core symptoms of fear and worry and, from a biological perspective, these can be linked to the neural circuitry of the amygdala (see Chapter 4). Anxiety and fear symptoms are regulated by an amygdala-centred circuit. The neurotransmitters that regulate these circuits include serotonin ($5HT_1$), GABA, glutamate, corticotrophin-releasing factor (CRF) and noradrenaline, among others.

Worry, by contrast, is regulated by part of the brain called the cortico-striatal thalamic-cortical (CSTC) loop. The circuits may be involved in all types of anxiety disorder but malfunction in

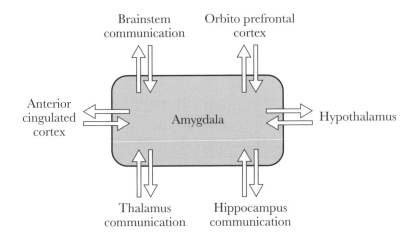

Figure 9.1: The amygdala communicates with different parts of the brain

different ways. For example, in GAD, the malfunctioning of these loops in the amygdala and CSTC may be persistent but not severe. In panic disorder, the malfunction may be intermittent, unexpected and catastrophic. In post-traumatic stress disorder (PTSD), the malfunction may be traumatic in origin or the circuits may be trapped in a redundant repetitive loop such as in OCD.

In addition to fear and worry, each anxiety subtype has its own specific symptoms. For example, people suffering from GAD may also experience irritability, muscle tension, arousal, fatigue, poor concentration and sleep disturbance.

Those suffering from panic disorder normally experience unexpected panic attacks and phobia or behavioural change, in addition to the core symptoms of fear and worry.

Symptoms of social anxiety disorder (also called social phobia) will normally include the expectation of panic attacks and phobic avoidance of the anxiety-provoking situations. In PTSD, the characteristic symptoms in addition to the core symptoms include the traumatic experience being relived, as well as worry about having other symptoms such as increased arousal, sleep difficulties such as nightmares, and avoidance behaviours.

Obsessive-compulsive disorders include the core symptoms of fear and worry, which tend to trigger obsessions and compulsions in an effort to reduce the worry and the obsessions themselves.

What differentiates one anxiety disorder from another is not necessarily the differences in anatomical localisation of the neurotransmitters regulating fear and worry; rather, it is the nature of the malfunction or dysfunction within these similar circuits in various anxiety disorders.

As a nurse you will not only come across people with the different kinds of anxiety we have just looked at, but also people with different physical illnesses that have given rise to anxiety. It is to these illnesses that we now turn.

Physical illnesses that may cause anxiety

As a nurse, you should be aware of the possibility that patients with the following conditions will also experience anxiety at some level:

- angina pectoris
- cardiac arrhythmias
- CNS degenerative disease
- Cushing's syndrome

- delirium
- hypoglycaemia
- hyperthyroidism
- Menière's disease

Now, before you read any further, try Activity 9.1.

Activity 9.1   *Critical thinking*

The experience of anxiety is common to most people and it can be beneficial.

- At what point does anxiety become a problematic emotion?
- Name the two symptoms that are common to all anxiety disorders.

An outline answer is provided at the end of the chapter.

The neurotransmitters involved in anxiety

In order to understand how medicines for anxiety work, you need to know about the neuro-transmitters involved in this condition. If you need to revise the anatomy involved, you may like to revisit Chapter 4.

Three main neurotransmitters involved in anxiety are GABA, serotonin and noradrenaline. As discussed in Chapter 4, GABA is the key inhibitory neurotransmitter and is involved in the reduction of activity of many neurons in the brain, including those found in the amygdala. When neurons are in an excited state, and fire rapidly, GABA binds to its own receptors and slows down neuronal activity to 'normal'. In other words, GABA works as the body's own natural anti-anxiety medicine. The anti-anxiety effect of GABA is increased if a benzodiazepine medicine binds to the GABA receptor. It must be noted that benzodiazepines only exert their therapeutic effect in the presence of the GABA neurotransmitter. If the neurotransmitter GABA is absent, benzodiazepines alone have no effect on neurons.

Earlier in this chapter we looked at the overlap in symptoms of depression and anxiety; not surprisingly, the neural circuitry of these two disorders also overlaps. For this reason, the neuro-transmitter serotonin is linked to both depression and anxiety symptoms. Serotonin is involved in the regulation of mood, impulse control, sleep, vigilance, eating, libido and cognitive functions such as memory and learning. It is also important in the modulation of anxiety and fear (Akimova et al., 2009). Preliminary findings suggest that it is the shortage of serotonin ($5HT_1$) in key areas of the brain such as the hippocampus, amygdala and anterior cingulated and raphe nuclei that probably causes these anxiety symptoms (Overstreet et al., 2003; Lanzenberger et al., 2007). This is why SSRIs (see Chapter 5) have become the first-line treatment for people with anxiety.

The third neurotransmitter that is involved in anxiety is noradrenaline, which is an excitatory neurotransmitter. Excessive output of noradrenaline in a part of the brainstem called the *locus coeruleus* can result in symptoms of anxiety such as fear, flashbacks, panic attacks, sweating and nightmares. It has been hypothesised that alpha$_1$ and beta$_1$ adrenergic receptors may be specifically involved in these reactions. Before you proceed to the next section, please try Activity 9.2.

Activity 9.2   *Critical thinking*

Chris is 26-year-old man who has an excessive fear of being in public places in case he vomits. Chris is aware that his fear is irrational, but nevertheless cannot stop himself worrying about vomiting in public places. Lately, his mood has been low because he is now socially restricted. He is not sure what medication he can benefit from and asks your advice.

- What is your likely advice to Chris?

An outline answer is provided at the end of the chapter.

Modern treatment of anxiety

When you have a patient suffering from an anxiety disorder, you need to work in partnership with the patient, taking a shared-decision approach. This relationship is the basis of successful care and management of the disorder. You should provide patients, and when appropriate the patient's family or carer, with all the relevant information they need, in a form they can understand. They will need to know about the nature and course of the problem, and the different treatment options available for anxiety. Medication may not be the only treatment option, as we shall see later in the chapter, but information on medication must include potential side effects. You should also provide patients, families and carers with information on self-help and support groups where appropriate. Before reading on, try Activity 9.3.

Activity 9.3   *Communication*

Use the internet to search for self-help groups and organisations that are located in your area and that help people suffering from anxiety. Make a list of the services they provide.

- If you were a patient who did not have internet access, how would this information be available to you?

An outline answer is provided at the end of the chapter.

Many patients with anxiety will choose psychological treatments. These include stress management, CBT, relaxation training, meditation, psychotherapy, and eye movement, desensitisation and reprocessing (EMDR) therapy. When medication is indicated, there are four main types of medicines available. But before we discuss these treatment options in more detail, you need to read the next case study.

Case study

Mavis is 28 years old and recently gave birth to a baby girl by Caesarean section after developing birth complications. After the birth of her child, she felt a little run down, but she put this down to tiredness and the difficult time she experienced giving birth. Gradually she began to worry about the health and safety of her newborn baby and the frequent trips she was making to the hospital. One day, when she was shopping for groceries in her local supermarket, she started to feel a little unwell, but pushed on with her shopping. By the time she got to the checkout, she was feeling uncomfortably stressed. She felt a tremendous sense of impending dread. Putting it down to tiredness, she continued unpacking her items from the trolley. That was when the first attack hit her. She couldn't breathe; her heart raced and felt like it would explode. Her legs almost crumpled under her and she badly wanted to run out of the shop, scream or grab somebody to help her. She didn't know what was happening to her. All she knew was that she felt like she was going to die. She grabbed the items she needed, threw them into a bag, somehow managed to toss some cash at the operator and fled from the shop. Back in the car she settled down a little, but she still felt terrible. She slowly drove home but, by the time she pulled into her driveway, she felt almost her old self again. She promptly forgot about the ordeal after a day or so. Unfortunately, this pattern of events repeated itself several times until she sought medical help. She was diagnosed with panic disorder and initially was prescribed and took clonazepam 2mg twice a day and fluoxetine 10mg once a day in the morning. The clonazepam was slowly tapered off after two weeks, while the fluoxetine was titrated up to a maintenance dose of 40mg a day. Mavis experienced relief of her symptoms within three days; however, she still worried excessively about the welfare of her child. After about nine weeks of treatment with fluoxetine she felt well enough to be able to attend the local anxiety management clinic.

Benzodiazepines

One of the drugs Mavis was given in the last case study, clonazepam, is a benzodiazepine, usually prescribed for epileptic seizures, but also useful in treating anxiety in the short term. There has been great concern about the addictive potential of benzodiazepines, which include diazepam, but in the short-term treatment of anxiety they may be prescribed. They are the most effective medicines available and are generally superior to psychological treatments, according to the American Psychiatric Association (APA) Task Force (1990). Once treatment continues beyond two weeks, however, both psychological and other medication treatments, particularly anti-depressants, become more effective (Tyrer et al., 1988). This is not only because other forms of treatment have a delayed onset of action, but also because tolerance develops to all the effects of benzodiazepines at a variable rate after repeated treatment. Benzodiazepines are therefore most appropriate for the emergency or planned short-term management of anxiety, such as the immediate relief of Mavis's panic attacks, and insomnia, rather than long-term use. From a risk perspective, benzodiazepines are very safe when taken singly, have few adverse effects in normal dosage and are liked by patients. This group as a whole is remarkably safe, although there can be additive effects with alcohol and other depressant medicines, particularly of the sedative-hypnotic type such as barbiturates.

Side effects of benzodiazepines

All benzodiazepines can induce psychomotor impairment. This particularly affects tasks that need coordination and vigilance, so you should warn patients of the risks of driving and operating machinery while on these medicines.

The risks with benzodiazepines increase when they are taken for four weeks or longer. This is mainly because of the risk of dependence, which is why Mavis was weaned off clonazepam after two weeks. People who become dependent suffer from discontinuation syndrome after reducing or stopping the medicine. The other major features of drug dependence (craving, medicine-seeking behaviour, escalation of dosage and marked tolerance) are not nearly so prevalent, although tolerance is now seen as a much greater problem than in the past. There is also some evidence that the more potent benzodiazepines, particularly those with a short elimination half-life, such as triazolam and lorazepam, may carry greater risks of dependence than others (Tyrer and Murphy, 1987), such as diazepam and clonazepam. It is for this reason that Mavis was prescribed clonazepam, a medicine with a relatively longer half-life and less addictive potential.

Symptoms of withdrawal normally begin within 24 hours of stopping a short-acting benzodi-azepine and up to six days after stopping a long-acting one. The terms 'rebound insomnia' and 'rebound anxiety' are sometimes used in the context of withdrawal reactions (Kales et al., 1978). However, there is no fundamental difference between the symptoms of rebound and those of withdrawal. It is just more common to use the term withdrawal when anti-anxiety medicines have been taken for a longer period.

Overdose from oral ingestion of benzodiazepines alone is generally not fatal. Most fatalities reported with this class of medicines tend to involve multiple medications, especially those medicines that depress the CNS, such as opiates, barbiturates and alcohol. Symptoms of benzodi-azepine overdose include drowsiness, confusion, somnolence, tiredness, impaired coordination, clumsiness in walking (ataxia) and slow reflexes. When multiple medications are implicated in benzodiazepine overdose, severe symptoms include difficulty breathing, slowed heart rate, low blood pressure, loss of coordination, and loss of consciousness leading to coma and, potentially, death. If you suspect an overdose, you should treat it as an emergency. The person should be taken to A&E for observation and treatment. You should bring the prescription bottle of medication and any other medication suspected in the overdose to the hospital, because the information on the prescription label can be helpful to the treating doctor.

An increasingly popular option in the treatment of anxiety is the use of antidepressants.

Antidepressants

Case study

Greg is a 40-year-old married artist with three children. He was diagnosed with pneumonia after a spell of feeling unwell. The doctor told him he was lucky to be alive and this made Greg very anxious that he has an illness that can potentially kill him. Although he recovered well from the pneumonia after a course of antibiotics, he started experiencing dizzy spells, sometimes vertigo, and weakness and he was sure his heart continued . . .

was weakening. Before long, his wife was rushing him to A&E because he was sure he was having a heart attack. The doctor examined him and pronounced his heart strong and healthy. Despite being pronounced fit, Greg deprived himself of sleep because he feared that, if he slept, he would have a heart attack and never wake up. This went on for so long that his behaviour was affecting his relationship with his family. He could not go too far away from home, where he felt safer. Greg continued to believe that there was something wrong with his heart, despite seeing a specialist who carried out thorough investigations and reassured him that there was nothing wrong. Greg was finally referred to a psychiatrist who diagnosed Greg with GAD. He was referred to a clinical psychologist for eight sessions of CBT and, in addition, his doctor prescribed sertraline 50mg to be taken in the morning. After about six weeks, Greg's condition improved so that he was able to go back to work part-time.

There is a growing body of evidence that antidepressants are effective in the treatment of primary anxiety disorders, as demonstrated in Greg's case. They have been extensively researched and SSRI antidepressants such as sertraline and/or benzodiazepines are commonly considered the first-line treatment, particularly for GAD. All antidepressants tend to work on the fear network by slowing down the action of the neurons.

Second in line in terms of effectiveness are the SNRI antidepressants, mirtazapine and MAOIs. If treatment is unsuccessful with these medications, TCAs can be used.

Antidepressants seem to be effective in reducing the symptoms of GAD in the medium to long term. However, their onset of action is about four to six weeks (Schmitt et al., 2005). We can see in the case study that Greg's fear and worry of having a heart attack diminished after six weeks of treatment with sertraline. Not all types of antidepressants are of proven effectiveness or of equal tolerability for a particular anxiety disorder, but there is now more evidence to inform selection. Before we discuss the next group of medicines used to treat anxiety, you need to try Activity 9.4.

Activity 9.4   *Critical thinking*

A patient on your ward is suffering from GAD and the doctor has prescribed fluoxetine 40mg to be taken at night. A staff nurse later approaches the doctor and asks her to correct the mistake.

- What do you think the error could be?

An outline answer is provided at the end of the chapter.

Azaspirones

Azaspirones are a group of medicines that work at the serotonin 5-HT_{1A} receptor and are used to treat patients suffering from GAD. One of the medicines, buspirone, was initially thought to possess antipsychotic properties, but this later proved to be incorrect. Further pharmacological and clinical evaluation of buspirone showed marked anxiolytic effects similar to those of diazepam (Goldberg, 1979). Since then, extensive neuropharmacological and clinical studies in animals and humans have demonstrated a unique anxiolytic profile for buspirone. In a systematic review of 36 studies, Chessick et al. (2006) found that, in general, azaspirones, and buspirone in particular, appear to be useful in the treatment of GAD especially for those participants who had not been on a benzodiazepine. This medication offers the benefit of reduced rumination and worry, without the problems of sedation and potential medicine dependence seen with benzodiazepines. It is not addictive and thus provides a treatment option for patients with GAD who are at risk of substance abuse. Recently, however, the use of certain anticonvulsants in the treatment of anxiety disorders has been increasing.

Anticonvulsants

On the basis of the hypothesis that anxiety results from excessive activation of the fear and worry circuits, it has been theorised that anticonvulsant medication can reduce this excitation in similar ways to which they reduce epileptic bursts. Researchers have investigated the use of various atypical anticonvulsants in the treatment of anxiety and, so far, the results for gabapentin, tiagabin, vigabatrin and levetiracetam have been modest (Ravindran and Stein, 2010). However, the use of pregabalin in the management of GAD has been widely investigated and it has been found to be effective. Patients tend to respond to pregabalin much quicker than to some antidepressants (Montgomery et al., 2006) and show an earlier response to treatment time than SNRI antidepressants such as venlafaxine.

Side effects of anticonvulsants

Common side effects of anticonvulsants used for anxiety disorders include sedation, dizziness, ataxia, memory impairment, confusion, blurred vision and abnormal coordination. For their management, see Chapter 6 on bipolar disorder. Next is an overview of some anxiety subtypes and their treatment and management.

Treatment and management of anxiety subtypes

Generalised anxiety disorder

Anxiety is often co-morbid with other illnesses such as depression or substance abuse. You should recommend psychotherapeutic strategies as the treatment of choice. Where this is not appropriate, benzodiazepines (diazepam, clonazepam, alprazolam) can be used. They have the advantage of providing rapid symptom relief, but unfortunately have no effect on the core symptom of worry. The elderly have difficulties in tolerating benzodiazepine adverse effects such as sedation and impaired physical coordination, therefore risking falls. For this reason benzodiazepines should be avoided in the elderly. Most patients with GAD respond well to 1–3mg/day of alprazolam or 1–2mg/day of clonazepam. TCAs cannot be used, due to their unfavourable side effects profile and their toxicity; they have been replaced by SSRIs and SNRIs as the first-line treatment. You need to monitor blood pressure in patients taking venlafaxine of doses above 300mg/day. Other effective anti-anxiety medicines are mirtazpine and SNRIs such as nefazodone. Buspirone, an azaspirone partial agonist, is effective in treating GAD without sedating the patient, nor does it cause dependence problems, but it does not relieve the physical symptoms. In some cases, atypical antipsychotics can be used as an adjunct treatment.

Obsessive-compulsive disorder

CBT can be effective and is a preferred psychotherapeutic option for OCD, providing a more lasting benefit than medicines. Other psychotherapeutic approaches are also effective. In any event, it is important to combine psychotherapeutic with psychopharmacological strategies to optimise treatment outcome. SSRIs are the first-line treatment and are usually initiated at low doses, approximately at half the initiation dose for depression treatment. You should inform patients that they may not experience a full therapeutic benefit for at least eight weeks and, in certain instances, this can be longer. If treatment is not effective, other options include switching to another SSRI, or to venlafaxine, duloxetine or clomipramine. It may be possible in some instances to augment antidepressant treatment with antipsychotics such as olanzapine or risperidone.

Social phobia

The mainstay treatment for social phobia is exposure-based therapy. In this regard, CBT is the therapy of choice and is best augmented with SSRIs such as paroxetine, sertraline or fluoxetine. As with OCD, venlafaxine is effective in the treatment of social phobia. Dose initiation is similar to that of OCD and many patients do not respond to treatment until they are receiving higher doses. If a patient fails to respond to treatment, switching to another SSRI should be considered. If this fails, then the SSRI can be augmented with a benzodiazepine, and clonazepam is a popular choice. If this also fails, then treatment can be augmented with the newer anticonvulsants such as pregabalin or gabapentin. Treatment can be continued for up to a year and medication can slowly be tapered off.

Post–traumatic stress disorder

As in other anxiety subtypes, psychotherapeutic approaches (especially EMDR) are augmented with psychopharmacological treatment for best results. During the acute stages, the combination of CBT and SSRIs is effective. Patients suffering from PTSD often experience depression and therefore the use of SSRIs is timely. SSRIs can make pre-existing anxiety worse but this is only temporary. To counter this, starting doses should be very low and you should warn patients that response time can be up to 12 weeks or longer. Many people with PTSD will still experience some symptoms despite treatment. For this reason, augmenting treatment is very common. For example, patients who continue to show impulsivity or lability of mood can be augmented with antipsychotics or mood stabilisers. In some situations, buspirone, mirtazapine or anticonvulsants can be effective augmentation.

Panic disorder

In acute situations, the priority is to control the frequency and intensity of symptoms. Benzodiazepines are particularly useful in people whose symptoms are so severe that they are unable to wait several weeks for antidepressants to take effect. An increasingly popular approach in the treatment of panic disorder is to concomitantly treat with benzodiazepines and anti-depressants. The benzodiazepine is gradually tapered off as the antidepressant is titrated up and used long term. In the medium term, a combination of CBT and antidepressants is preferred. Also, antidepressants may be preferred if a patient is unsure about CBT or cannot invest enough time in therapy. With regard to the elderly, the use of antidepressants may be preferred to benzodiazepines because of the difficulty the elderly have in tolerating the adverse effects of benzodiazepines. Because panic disorders are typically chronic illnesses, treatment is usually for up to nine months after symptoms have remitted.

Common management errors to avoid

When a patient presents with anxiety, it is important to ask the patient for his or her full medical history, as anxiety could be secondary to a pre-existing physical illness. In such cases, it is important to treat the underlying physical condition. Also, always take note of any current medication the patient may be taking as some medications cause anxiety. Avoid using TCAs in the elderly because of their adverse effects (especially antimuscarinic effects). Also avoid using benzodiazepines in this population as these medicines can cause confusion and coordination impairment. SSRIs should not be administered at night as they have a tendency to cause sleep disturbance, and benzodiazepines should be avoided in patients who have a concurrent substance abuse problem. Psychotherapeutic approaches are quite effective in the treatment of anxiety, so it is important to offer these therapies in tandem with medication for maximum effect.

What the patient and carers need to know

- Normally, both fear and anxiety can be helpful, helping us to avoid dangerous situations, making us alert and giving us the motivation to deal with problems. However, if the feelings become too strong or go on for too long, they can stop us from doing the things we want to and can make our lives miserable.
- Talking about the problem to friends or family can be beneficial and finding ways of learning to relax can help control anxiety and tension. Everything from books and video tapes to seeking professional advice can offer an insight on how to relax. Self-help groups and psychotherapy are other options that may help patients to come to terms with the reasons for their anxiety.
- Medication can play a role if the other options are not appropriate. The most common medications are benzodiazepines, buspirone and atypical anticonvulsants.
- Patients prescribed benzodiazepines should not drive or operate machinery.
- Patients prescribed SSRIs should not stop the medication abruptly as this will cause discontinuation syndrome. They should be informed that antidepressants can take up to six weeks or longer to work. Also, if a patient misses an antidepressant dose, he or she should be

advised to take it as soon as possible within two to three hours of the scheduled dose. If it is close to the next scheduled dose, they should skip the missed dose and continue on the regular dosing schedule. Patients should not take double doses. Most antidepressants can be taken with or without food.

- You should advise the patient to store the medication in its originally labelled, light-resistant container, away from heat and moisture. Heat and moisture may precipitate breakdown of the medication, and it may lose its therapeutic effect.

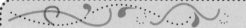

Chapter summary

Anxiety as a disorder has existed for a long time and people who suffer from this condition typically experience feelings of apprehension, fear, physical tension, irritation and worry. There are several subtypes of anxiety, namely generalised anxiety disorder, phobias, obsessive compulsive disorder, panic disorder and post-traumatic stress disorder. Each subtype has its own characteristics and symptoms that require different treatment. Psychotherapeutic approaches to treatment are preferred for anxiety disorders, so it is important to offer these therapies in tandem with medication for maximum effect. SSRI antidepressants are the first medicine of choice and other classic antidepressants are also effective. Benzodiazepines are also useful, particularly for GAD and during the acute stages of panic disorder. Their use in the elderly, however, should be restricted because of adverse side effects.

Activities: brief outline answers

Activity 9.1 When anxiety becomes a problem (page 174)

Anxiety is normal, and in normal cases it allows us to overcome obstacles by preparing ourselves. However, it becomes a clinical problem when the individual cannot function normally as a result. Fear and worry are common to all anxiety disorders.

Activity 9.2 Fear of vomiting in public (page 175)

Chris is showing symptoms of fear, anxiety and depression. SSRIs are probably a good option because they act on the fear and worry loop. SSRIs will be able to relieve the symptoms of depression that Chris is experiencing.

Activity 9.3 Self-help groups (page 175)

If patients and relatives have no internet at home, you could advise them to use the internet in libraries or internet cafés. Alternatively, you could advise patients to seek information about local self-help groups from their GPs.

Activity 9.4 Fluoxetine (page 178)

Fluoxetine, an SSRI, causes sleep disturbance and it is best taken in the morning rather than at night. By contrast, tricyclic medicines such as amitriptyline cause sedation and therefore are best taken at night rather than in the morning.

Further reading

Clark, DA and Beck, A (2009) *Cognitive Therapy for Anxiety Disorders: Science and practice*. London: Guilford Press.

A useful book that deals with practical aspects of CBT for anxiety.

Wells, A (1997) *Cognitive Therapy of Anxiety Disorders: A practice manual and conceptual guide*. Chichester: Wiley.

This is a good guide for those practising CBT for anxiety.

Useful websites

www.anxietyuk.org.uk

Anxiety UK is a national registered charity for agoraphobia and those affected by other anxiety disorders. It is run by sufferers and ex-sufferers, supported by a high-profile medical advisory panel and provides information, support and understanding via an extensive range of services, including one-to-one therapy.

www.social-anxiety.org.uk

This site aims to provide information for people with social anxiety and related issues. It has links to further information and acts as a central hub for those with social anxiety problems in the UK.

Chapter 10
Management and treatment of substance misuse disorders

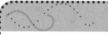

NMC Standards for Pre-registration Nursing Education

This chapter will address the following competencies:

Domain 1: Professional values

Field standard for competence

Mental health nurses must work with people of all ages using values-based mental health frameworks. They must use different methods of engaging people, and work in a way that promotes positive relationships focused on social inclusion, human rights and recovery, that is, a person's ability to live a self-directed life, with or without symptoms, that they believe is meaningful and satisfying.

NMC Essential Skills Clusters

This chapter will address the following ESCs:

Cluster: Medicines management

36. People can trust the newly registered graduate nurse to ensure safe and effective practice in medicines management through comprehensive knowledge of medicines, their actions, risks and benefits.

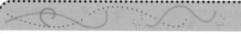

Chapter aims

By the end of this chapter, you should be able to:

- understand the mechanism that underpins the reward system in substance misuse;
- outline the medicines used for alcohol abuse, their modes of action and side effects;
- explain the medicines used for opiate withdrawal, their modes of action and side effects;
- appreciate the common errors to avoid in the treatment of substance misuse;
- communicate necessary information to patients who misuse substances.

Introduction

Case study

Darren has just been released from prison where he was serving a five-year sentence for armed robbery. He uses cocaine, cannabis and heroin. Before Darren became a polydrug user, he was employed as a physical fitness instructor in the army. He started using drugs after the death of his wife in a car crash in which he was the driver. His first experience of smoking cocaine was a feeling of extreme euphoria and pleasure, which contrasted greatly with the low mood he was then experiencing. However, the feeling of euphoria and pleasure did not last long and soon he was looking for cocaine to gratify his need. In a very short period, Darren was addicted to drugs and this had a dramatic effect on his life. He lost his job and many friends deserted him. He turned to crime to finance his habit and therefore came into conflict with the law. He has been in prison more than once for crimes related to drug abuse. He has tried to give up drugs several times but has not succeeded. While in prison, he made several attempts on his life. His probation officer has recommended that Darren attends a drug treatment centre as a condition of release, which he has gratefully accepted.

The use of psychoactive substances is common in people with mental and behavioural disorders. The most commonly used substances are tobacco, alcohol, opiates, cannabis, cocaine, sedatives and volatile solvents. These substances induce a variety of mental and behavioural states that range from intoxication and harmful use (abuse) dependence to aggression and co-morbid psychiatric disorders (dual diagnosis). 'Habitual use' of these substances can cause physical or mental health problems, while 'substance dependence' is diagnosed when the use of substances becomes compulsive, uncontrollable and associated with physiological withdrawal symptoms. Also, the sole pursuit of people who are dependent on these substances is to use them, despite their experience of serious harm to themselves or others.

The use of alcohol is the most common and it is estimated that, in the UK, 24 per cent of adult men and 13 per cent of adult women drink in a hazardous or harmful way (NICE, 2009c). The prevalence of drug abuse and dependence ranges from 0.4 to 4 per cent, and this includes heroin and cocaine-use disorders (0.25 per cent). Injecting drugs is associated with a high risk globally for contracting blood-borne infections, including hepatitis B, hepatitis C and HIV (Murray and Lopez, 1996). Overall, the highest rates of substance misuse occur during late adolescence and early adulthood. In those who will eventually have a substance misuse disorder, the pattern of use evolves from 'experimentation' to overt substance abuse fairly rapidly.

Controversy remains over the view that substance use disorders are not medical disorders but are expressions of lifestyle or, at worst, of criminal behaviours by people who inflict these problems on themselves. Irrespective of the moral arguments, there can be no doubt that serious physical and mental health problems result from the use of these substances. Moreover, there is sufficient evidence that susceptibility to substance misuse has an inheritable genetic basis, as demonstrated by a recent review (Muller et al., 2010). Therefore, many drug abusers do not choose this way of life. Psychological factors also contribute to the risk of substance abuse, so patients suffering from depression and anxiety, and individuals who tend to be thrill seekers or who are prone to agitation and aggression, are at a greater risk of abusing substances.

While the use of substances arguably contributes to the propensity for aggression and reck-lessness, there is evidence that these traits in substance abusers date back to childhood and therefore pre-date the onset of substance abuse. It is also argued that the substance abuse itself may be an attempt to self-medicate for these behavioural traits or other psychiatric disorders. This is a good reason to ask a patient with any psychological disorder, such as depression or anxiety, whether or not they have found anything that seems to help their condition.

To better understand treatments for substance misuse disorders, it is necessary for you to understand the mechanism underlying addictive behaviour; the dopamine theory of reward offers a plausible explanation.

The dopamine theory of reward

In psychology, a reward is a process that reinforces behaviour. In other words, it is something that, when offered, causes a behaviour to increase in intensity. Also, rewards induce learning and positive emotions. Natural rewards include eating, drinking, sex and fighting.

The *reward circuit*, also referred to as the dopamine mesolimbic system, is generally accepted as the common pathway of reward and reinforcement involved in substance misuse. This pathway is also referred to as the 'pleasure centre' and dopamine has been labelled the 'pleasure neurotransmitter'. Please refer to Chapter 7 on the treatment of psychosis, and to Figure 7.1, for details.

An increase in dopamine levels in the mesolimbic (reward) system produces a pleasurable feeling. There are many natural ways to trigger the release of dopamine, such as passing an examination, listening to music you enjoy, watching a funny movie, eating food, drinking or having sex. Conversely, dopamine neurons are depressed when the expected reward is omitted. In nature, we learn to repeat behaviours that lead to maximising rewards. Dopamine is therefore believed to provide a teaching signal to parts of the brain responsible for acquiring new behaviours.

To be able to produce these feelings of joy or 'natural highs', the mesolimbic pathway is regulated by an array of chemicals that includes the brain's own natural drugs, such as opiates (endorphins), cannabis (anandamide) and nicotine (acetylcholine). An increase in these natural drugs in the brain will result in the increase of dopamine levels in the limbic region, causing feelings of euphoria.

Case study

Kevin is a 24-year-old man who was transferred to hospital from prison where he was serving a sentence for multiple counts of burglary. Kevin started smoking cannabis when he was 15 years old and he very quickly moved to taking crack cocaine. He soon discovered he had to increase his intake of cocaine to get the same level of satisfaction as before. For Kevin, this meant he had to steal from houses to finance his drug habit, which is why he went to prison.

With respect to drugs of abuse, nearly all drugs, directly or indirectly, target the brain's mesolimbic system by flooding the circuit with dopamine. The overstimulation of this system, which normally responds to natural behaviours linked to survival (such as eating and drinking), produces euphoric effects and this reaction sets in motion a pattern that 'teaches' people to repeat the behaviour of abusing these drugs. As a person continues to abuse drugs, the brain responds by adapting to the overwhelming surges in dopamine by producing less dopamine or by reducing the number of dopamine receptors in the reward circuit. This lessens the impact of dopamine on the reward circuit therefore reducing the abuser's ability to enjoy the drugs, as in Kevin's case. This decrease compels those addicted to keep abusing drugs in order to attempt to bring their dopamine function back to 'normal'. But they may now require larger amounts of the drug than they first did to achieve the dopamine high and this effect is known as *tolerance*. Most people who abuse drugs resort to committing crime to finance their drug-taking habit, which brings them to the attention of law enforcement agencies.

Non-conscious or *conditioned learning* is a type of learning in which a stimulus acquires the capacity to induce an unconscious response that was originally induced by a different stimulus. Substances of abuse facilitate conditioned learning, which leads the user to experience uncontrollable cravings when they see a place or person they associate with the drug experience, even when the drug itself is not available. Brain imaging studies of drug-addicted individuals show changes in areas of the brain that are critical to judgement, decision-making, learning and memory, and behaviour control (Cosgrove, 2010). Together, these changes can drive an abuser to seek out and take drugs compulsively despite adverse consequences. There is a wide variety of medications used in the treatment of substance misuse disorder and these vary according to the type of substance being abused, as well as patient choice and motivation. In spite of this variety, their use has a common theoretical base and we will briefly review these theories.

Care and management approaches

The core value or guiding principle for the treatment and management of those who misuse substances is that such persons have the same entitlement to health and social care as other patients. It is therefore your responsibility, as it of all other healthcare professionals involved, to provide for their general health and social needs in addition to their drug-related problems. The care and management of people with substance misuse disorders can be divided into two stages:

1. the detoxification stage;
2. the rehabilitation stage.

The key to a successful detoxification regime is good preparation. Before you read further, you need to try Activity 10.1.

Activity 10.1   *Critical thinking*

You receive a phone call from one of your patients who drinks heavily, informing you that he wishes to 'end it all'. He says he has not been drinking for a day and feels irritable and

---

continued . . .

sweaty. He is not sure whether he should continue to drink alcohol or not and he needs help to 'sort his life out'.

• How would you respond to this call?

An outline answer is provided at the end of the chapter.

Your first responsibility as a nurse is to bring the patient to a point of readiness to change their substance misuse behaviour by applying the popular stages of behaviour change model (Prochaska and DiClemente, 1984b) (see Figure 3.2 on page 77). This means that the patient has to reach at least the contemplation stage. At this stage, patients are sufficiently well motivated to make a sustained effort to change. In other words, they have reached a good-quality decision to change, because they feel physically unwell, are under pressure from family or work, or simply feel the need for a temporary break from their substance misuse. Patients need to be given accurate information about what to expect during detoxification as information-giving is likely to reduce the severity of the withdrawal and increase adherence (Phillips et al., 1986). In the course of discussion with the patient, it is often useful to map out a timetable for the week in which detoxification will take place and for the following week, as this will bring up a number of important issues, such as work commitments, childcare arrangements, transport difficulties and personal support.

It is important to understand the cause of the problem and to assess its consequences in order to establish the patient's strengths and weaknesses. If you carry out a good assessment, you will be able to formulate a good overall care and medicines management plan. You should provide care that is evidence-based, including harm-reduction approaches (DH, 1999). Another aspect that promotes good care is effective key working.

Effective key working

The NICE guidelines (2010) stipulate that, in order to ensure that a person gets full benefit from care, you should adopt effective key working as it helps to deliver high-quality outcomes for people who misuse substances. If you are a key worker, you have a central role in coordinating a care plan and building a therapeutic alliance with the patient, as the benefits of any treatment approach in substance misuse can only be realised within the context of properly coordinated care. Also, you should take into account of patient's needs and preferences. People who misuse substances should have the opportunity to make informed decisions about their care and treatment, in partnership with you. If a patient does not have the capacity to make decisions, you should use the Mental Capacity Act 2005 to guide you (see Chapter 2). You should also ensure good communication between yourself and the patient. Any information you give to the patient regarding their treatment should be supported by evidence and it should be tailored to the patient's needs and culturally appropriate. In addition, always ensure that any information you give is accessible to people with additional needs such as sensory or learning disabilities, and to people who do not speak or read English. If the patient is in agreement, families and carers should have the opportunity to be involved in decisions about care and management and will also need information and support. As alcohol is the most widely used substance, we will now discuss this in more detail.

Alcohol

The production and use of alcohol is common in many cultures and may go back to ancient Egyptian and Mesopotamian civilisations. Alcohol is a CNS depressant that shares many pharmacological properties with the non-benzodiazepine sedative-hypnotics and barbiturates. It affects the CNS in a dose-dependent fashion (the larger the quantity, the more the effect), producing sedation that progresses to sleep, unconsciousness, coma, surgical anaesthesia and, finally, fatal respiratory depression and cardiovascular collapse. Alcohol intake increases the body's own naturally occurring opiates and this may be responsible for the euphoria experienced. It also affects several neurotransmitter systems in the brain, including GABA, glutamate and dopamine.

It is probably the most studied substance, mainly because it is the most abused. It is associated with dependence, abuse, withdrawal, intoxication, delirium, dementia, amnesia, delusions, hallucinations, mood disorder, anxiety disorder and sexual dysfunction. Psychiatric symptoms are very common in people who misuse alcohol, but most of these symptoms subside within weeks of stopping alcohol. Schizophrenia, depression and personality disorder are the most common disorders associated with alcohol misuse. Since alcohol is a depressant, it tends to produce symptoms of depression during intoxication and anxiety symptoms during withdrawal and abstinence (Preston et al., 2008).

The goals of treatment should normally include suppression of symptoms and the prevention of complications that arise from abstinence. In general, less than half of alcoholic patients report withdrawal symptoms. In most cases these symptoms do not require intervention, often disappearing within two to seven days of the last drink. Patients should be considered for detoxification if they:

- are severely dependent on alcohol;
- have a history of delirium tremens and alcohol withdrawal seizures;
- have a poor social support network;
- have poor physical health that includes cardiac, pulmonary, hepatic, kidney or cardiovascular diseases;
- have cognitive and memory impairment;
- have psychiatric co-morbidity (depression, psychosis or personality disorder).

You should be aware that the manifestation of alcohol withdrawal tends to differ from person to person but usually occurs within 6–24 hours after the last drink. Symptoms can include mild insomnia, increases in blood pressure and pulse rate, tremors, **hyper-reflexia**, irritability, anxiety and depression. *Alcohol withdrawal syndrome* (AWS) can be a life-threatening condition affecting some alcohol-dependent patients who discontinue or decrease their alcohol consumption too suddenly. The symptoms of severe AWS may progress to more complicated forms characterised by delirium tremens, seizures and coma. In these forms, cardiac arrest and death may occur in 5–10 per cent of patients (Schuckit et al., 1995). For this reason, it is important for you to systematically assess the level or severity of dependency in an individual, preferably using a clinical rating scale.

There are many rating scales for assessment of alcohol withdrawal but the best known and most extensively studied is the Clinical Institute Withdrawal Assessment – Alcohol (CIWA – A) and a shortened version, the CIWA – A revised (CIWA – Ar), which is a carefully refined list of 10 signs

Symptom severity	0	1	2	3	4	5	6	7
Agitation								
Anxiety								
Auditory disturbances								
Clouding of sensorium								
Headache								
Nausea/vomiting								
Paroxysmal sweats								
Tactile disturbances								
Tremor								
Visual disturbances								

Table 10.1: The CIWA – Ar scale

and symptoms (Wiehl et al., 1994); each item scores a minimum of 0 and maximum of 7 (see Table 10.1). The CIWA – Ar has added usefulness because high scores, in addition to indicating severe withdrawal, are also predictive of the development of seizures and delirium.

Total scores on the CIWA – Ar of less than 8 to10 indicate minimal to mild withdrawal. Scores of 8 to 15 indicate moderate withdrawal (marked autonomic arousal); and scores of 15 or more indicate severe withdrawal. A study of the CIWA – Ar predicted that those with a score of over 15 were at increased risk of severe alcohol withdrawal and the higher the score the greater the risk. However, you should be aware that some patients can suffer complications in spite of low scores, if left untreated. You should always explain procedures fully to the patient and answer any questions. As usual, always seek consent before carrying out procedures. An assessment is usually followed by a detoxification regime, and we now look at an example.

Alcohol detoxification

The process of alcohol detoxification requires that alcohol be eliminated from the body and that any withdrawal or other symptoms that are bound to occur are treated medically or psychologically, or both. You should be aware that AWS can be quite distressing and can even become fatal if the addiction to alcohol is very severe. The patient needs to be an inpatient for at least a week to remain under constant supervision, as the sudden cessation of alcohol consumption can lead to other symptoms that require medical intervention. Some patients who undergo the alcohol detoxification process may suffer from hallucinations, delirium tremens and even convulsions, which if not immediately attended to can be fatal.

Detoxification regime

- You should start by completing a CIWA on admission to the ward and then eight-hourly for 24 hours.
- Record vital signs such as blood pressure, pulse, temperature, oxygen concentration and peak flow. On admission, determine blood alcohol concentration (BAC) using a breathalyser.
- Keep recording vital signs every four hours and call the doctor if the patient's diastolic blood pressure is greater than 120mmHg, or systolic blood pressure is greater than 180mmHg.

There are medicines available that can be used to minimise these symptoms, but the administration of these has to be very properly controlled and monitored, so that any side effects are quickly treated. Initial dosages of such medicines are always high, but are gradually decreased during the detoxification programme. At present, benzodiazepines are the medicines of choice in the treatment of AWS, since they have proven their efficacy in ameliorating symptoms and decreasing the risk of seizures and delirium tremens. Benzodiazepines are usually administered for the first seven days of a detoxification programme.

Benzodiazepines

Theoretically, any benzodiazepine can be used for detoxification. The choice depends on the patient's circumstances. For example, if a patient has liver disease, it may be appropriate to prescribe a short-acting benzodiazepine such as lorazepam or oxazepam. Longer-acting benzodiazepines may be appropriate for those prone to seizures, but may not be appropriate in the elderly. In people with mild dependence, very small amounts of chlordiazepoxide can be used, or the condition can be managed without medication. In moderate dependence, larger doses of chlordiazepoxide may be required and this can be up to 40mg per day. This dose can be slowly reduced to 0 over a period of five to seven days. Severe alcohol withdrawal requires even larger doses of chlordiazepoxide under inpatient treatment. In most cases, it not unusual for doctors to prescribe a benzodiazepine immediately as a single dose (a *stat dose*) after the patient has been seen by the doctor during the admission process. This stat dose is usually based on the severity of the symptoms at the time and the concentration of alcohol shown by the breathalyser. In most cases, doctors tend to prescribe this stat dose as 5–50mg of chlordiazepoxide (Taylor et al., 2007). In extreme cases where a patient is experiencing severe alcohol withdrawal symptoms, chlordiazepoxide doses of up to 250mg have been known, but this is only under the supervision of a specialist.

After the initial period of assessment, which last for 24 hours, a reducing regimen of chlordiazepoxide is normally instituted and this can last between five and seven days. The medicine can be given in divided doses with higher evening and night doses to aid sleeping. In most cases, the dose is reduced by about 6 per cent of the original dose, but a longer period of reduction might be necessary, particularly for those patients suffering delirium tremens. During the withdrawal stage, and particularly after the administration of chlordiazepoxide, you need continually to observe and record the patient's physical and mental state. If necessary, you need to rate withdrawal symptoms using the CIWA and record vital signs every four hours. Before you proceed further with this chapter, try Activity 10.2.

| Activity 10.2 | *Critical thinking* |

You have been asked to carry out admission procedures on a 45-year-old man who suffers from depression. During the admission interview, he appears irritable and forgetful and shows fine tremors. He informs you that he has been drinking two bottles of whisky a day.

- In light of this information, what might you incorporate in the admission procedure?

An outline answer is provided at the end of the chapter.

Vitamin supplementation

It is common practice for all patients going through an alcohol withdrawal programme to be offered thiamine (vitamin B1) to prevent Wernicke's encephalopathy (WE) and this is normally given for about five days, followed by oral vitamin B compound. Parenteral thiamine is given in extreme alcohol withdrawal cases because oral thiamine is poorly absorbed in those who have been drinking heavily.

Long-term relapse prevention

The long-term care of people with alcohol misuse problems should be carried out in the community where benzodiazepines have no place beyond the detoxification stage. As previously mentioned, the treatment plan should be customised to meet individual needs. You should note that the use of medicines to treat substance-related problems without psychosocial intervention sends the wrong message to the patient. The substance abuser already leans heavily on substances to either escape or solve problems and we should not collude in the dependence on substances to solve all problems. Nevertheless, medicines do play an important role in recovery.

Several medicines have been licensed for the treatment of alcohol dependence in the long term. To understand how these medicines work, we need to understand how alcohol exerts its effects. The action of alcohol on the opiate synapse will result in the release of dopamine into the reward circuit (see 'The dopamine theory of reward' on pages 186–7). Alcohol may do this by acting directly on the μ (mu) opiate receptors or by releasing natural opiates, such as enkelphalin, that stimulate the release of dopamine in the reward circuit.

Case study

Chris has been drinking heavily for over eight years since the break-up of his marriage. He accepts that his drinking has caused further problems in his life and wants to stop drinking. Having made several attempts to give up drinking in the past, Chris is aware of the difficulties of abstaining from alcohol. His doctor suggested that he could consider a medicine called naltrexone, which works by reducing his ability to enjoy alcohol. He was happy to try this medicine.

Medicines such as naltrexone work by blocking opiate receptors, therefore limiting dopamine release into the reward system. By limiting the amount of dopamine in the reward system, the medicine naltrexone effectively blocks the enjoyment of drinking. The usual dose of naltrexone for alcohol dependence is 50mg daily, although a few patients may require only 25mg daily. The use of naltrexone is a good example of *interference therapy*. Another alcohol treatment takes the form of *aversion therapy* and this is best exemplified by the use of disulfiram.

Disulfiram

Case study

Jenny is 33 years old and suffers from depression. She was physically and sexually abused as a young girl and has been drinking alcohol heavily since she was 15. She currently drinks two to three bottles of spirits a day. She has abstained from drinking on several occasions in the past but this never really lasted. Although she is determined to stop drinking, she is worried about the possibility of relapsing. After a discussion with her doctor, she has agreed to have a medicine called Antabuse (disulfiram) implanted in the lining of her stomach to help her abstain.

In aversion therapy, the medication will make the effects of using alcohol extremely uncomfortable. One such medicine is disulfiram, which discourages the patient from drinking by producing an aversive reaction if the patient is exposed to alcohol; however, when a person abstains, the medicine has minimal effects. Maintenance doses can range anywhere from 125mg to 500mg daily, with the average dose being 250mg daily.

Disulfiram works by inhibiting an enzyme in the liver called *aldehyde dehydrogenase*, which is responsible for breaking down alcohol **metabolites** called aldehydes. This allows aldehydes to accumulate in the body. The resulting increase in aldehydes causes severe facial flushing, throbbing headache, nausea and vomiting, chest pain, palpitations, tachycardia, weakness, dizziness, blurred vision, confusion and hypotension. Severe reactions include myocardial infarction, congestive heart failure, cardiac arrhythmia, respiratory depression and convulsions; death can occur, particularly in vulnerable individuals.

A disulfiram reaction can occur up to two weeks after therapy has been discontinued, but the time of risk is usually four to seven days. Even the small amount of alcohol contained in mouthwashes, certain foodstuffs and medicines can cause a reaction. Although rare, a potentially fatal idiosyncratic liver toxicity reaction can occur with disulfiram. Therefore, baseline liver function tests should be obtained and the patient monitored for liver toxicity (hepatoxicity) by symptoms and by repeating the liver function tests at certain intervals. If a patient opts for disulfiram, you should explain all the possible risks involved so they can make an informed choice, including side effects and the effects of drinking alcohol while on the medication.

Most common side effects of disulfiram are transient, but occasionally patients may experience skin eruptions that can be controlled with an antihistamine. Another medicine that is used in the long-term management of people with alcohol misuse problems is acamprosate.

Acamprosate

Acamprosate is a synthetic compound that is structurally similar to the inhibitory neuro-transmitter GABA and is neither a sedative nor an anxiolytic. More importantly, acamprosate is not addictive nor has reinforcing effects on humans. Unlike naltrexone, acamprosate does not reduce the rewarding effects of alcohol; nor does it precipitate aversive negative symptoms when co-ingested with alcohol, as with disulfiram. Because withdrawal of alcohol following chronic usage can lead to excessive glutamate activity and reduced GABA activity, acamprosate appears to work by stimulating the GABA receptors and decreasing excitation at the glutamate (NMDA) receptors. Acamprosate has been shown to suppress alcohol-stimulated increase of dopamine in part of the reward circuit called the *nucleus acumbens*. It is supplied as an enteric-coated tablet for oral administration. Patients should be advised to swallow the tablets whole and not to crush, cut or chew them. A dose of two 333mg enteric-coated tablets three times a day with meals is recommended by the manufacturer to aid adherence. Acamprosate therapy should be started as soon as possible after alcohol detoxification to maintain abstinence as part of a comprehensive psycho-social treatment programme. For patients with moderate renal impairment, the recommended dose is one 333mg tablet three times a day. Patients with severe renal impairment should not receive acamprosate therapy. As stated earlier, acamprosate is not metabolised by the liver to any known extent. Dosage adjustments are not necessary for older patients unless they have renal impairment. Acamprosate is well tolerated, with diarrhoea being the most common adverse effect. In many cases, the care and management of people with alcohol misuse problems is similar for those with drug dependence, to which we now turn.

Care and management of drug abuse and dependence

As with alcohol-related problems, the treatment of people with drug problems requires that you consider the individual in their personal and social contexts, while being mindful of the complex interaction of these factors and how they affect the individual. Therefore, treatment will typically include social, psychological, educational and pharmacological therapies. Again, as with alcohol misuse, treatment should result in recovery and a health benefit. Consequently, the goals of treatment should be tailored to the healthcare needs of the individual; with many patients treatment will include abstinence as an explicit objective, while with other patients intermediate goals, such as reduction of harmful injecting, may be more realistic and achievable.

There are many different types of drugs that people misuse and each of these classes may require different pharmacological approaches. The types we will look at are the stimulants and opiates.

Stimulants

Scenario

Obeng is a 26-year-old man who has been treated for a psychotic disorder since he dropped out of university two years ago. At the time, he was using cannabis regularly, but soon moved to crack cocaine because it was

continued . . .

> *cheap and easily available. He particularly enjoyed the intense pleasurable feeling that he derived from the drug. He was admitted to hospital following deterioration in his mental state and his mother stated that he was spending most of his time looking for drugs. Lately, he has not been able to get any drugs because he cannot find the money to finance his habit. On admission to hospital, Obeng has stated that he feels irritable and depressed.*

Stimulants are a group of drugs that people tend to become dependent on or addicted to. They include cocaine, cannabis, hallucinogens, ecstasy and amphetamines. Unfortunately, there are no effective medications for treating stimulant dependence, despite trials of several agents (de Lima et al., 2002).

Stimulant drugs such as amphetamines, cocaine and ecstasy do not produce a major physiological withdrawal syndrome and can be stopped abruptly, such as with Obeng. However, people who have regularly used stimulant drugs may experience insomnia and depressed mood when they stop taking them. Like stimulants, hallucinogenic drugs such as LSD do not produce a physical withdrawal syndrome and can also be stopped abruptly. Care and management involves calming and reassuring the patient until the effects wear off. Occasionally, oral diazepam (10–20mg) may be needed to help calm the patient, and in severe cases where symptoms do persist, antipsychotic medication may be needed.

If a patient is experiencing low mood, antidepressant medicines can be used, but many stimulant users just need advice regarding the likely symptoms and reassurance that they will pass. In Obeng's case, you should assess the severity of his depression and look out for suicidal ideation, which will require close observation. There is no recognised role for substitute prescribing in the management of stimulant withdrawal.

Rarely, cocaine overdose can result in cardiovascular complications, including arrhythmia, hypertension and cardiac ischaemia. Seizures and hyperpyrexia can also occur. In such cases, treatment is supportive as there are no specific drugs used to reverse the effect of cocaine. Some people experience severe distress during or after use of hallucinogenic drugs and may need symptomatic treatment (such as a brief course of a benzodiazepine to reduce anxiety) as well as a safe place to be while the experience passes.

Opiates

Opiates act as neurotransmitters in neurons that arise from the ventral tegmental area (VTA) to the nucleus accumbens in the brain. The body's own natural opiates, such as endorphins or enkephalins, which are stored in the opiate neurons, act on a variety of opiate receptors that include the mu (μ), delta (δ) and kappa (κ) receptors. Opiate drugs of abuse, such as heroin, also act in a similar manner by mimicking the body's natural opiates (endorphins or enkephalins) particularly at μ receptors. They induce a very intense but brief euphoria, sometimes called a 'rush', followed by a profound sense of tranquillity that may last several hours, followed by drowsiness, mood swings, mental clouding, apathy and slowed motor movements. In overdose, opiates act as respiratory depressants and can induce coma. When given chronically, opiates easily cause tolerance and dependence.

As with alcohol, one of the first obstacles you may face as a nurse is how to assess opiate withdrawal symptoms. There are clear advantages in using a rating instrument that provides accurate and clinically relevant measurement, such as the shortened version of the Opiate Withdrawal Scale (Gossop, 1990). This scale (see Table 10.2) provides a satisfactory and valid measure of the distress experienced by people withdrawing from opiates; it is a straightforward, clinically useful and easy-to-use instrument that takes less than a minute to complete.

The most commonly selected opioid for detoxification is methadone, because it is more effective and well absorbed after oral administration. It has a relatively long half-life, so once- or twice-daily doses give an extended duration of cover against the more extreme aspects of withdrawal (Stahl, 2008). Opioid dependence should be confirmed by evidence of usage such as positive urine results for opioids, recent sites of injection (depending on the route), and objective signs and symptoms of withdrawal, including nausea, stomach cramps, insomnia, muscular tension, muscle spasm/twitching, aches and pains. Opioid withdrawal reactions are very uncomfortable but are not life-threatening, and it is important to ask the patient when they had their last dose, as withdrawal symptoms tend to peak at around 32–72 hours after the last dose of opiates was taken. In general, symptoms tend to subside after five days.

As with anyone suffering from a mental health disorder, the issue of importance in treating with opioid withdrawal symptoms is not so much treating the disease state as treating the individual. You should take account of a patient's emotional and spiritual condition as this plays an important part in the recovery process. During the process of obtaining informed consent from the patient, you should provide detailed information about the detoxification procedure and any possible risks. You should also explain about the physical and psychological aspects of opioid

Symptom	None	Mild	Moderate	Severe
Feeling sick				
Stomach cramps				
Muscle spasms/twitching				
Feeling of coldness				
Heart pounding				
Muscular tension				
Aches and pains				
Yawning				
Runny eyes				
Insomnia/problems sleeping				

Table 10.2: The shortened Opiate Withdrawal Scale

withdrawal such as the duration and intensity of symptoms, and how these may be managed, including the use of non-medicinal approaches. It is important that you explain to the patient that there will be loss of tolerance to opiods following detoxification and an ensuing increased risk of overdose and death from illicit drug use that may be worsened by the use of alcohol or benzodiazepines. You should emphasise the importance of continued support, as well as psychosocial and appropriate pharmacological interventions, to maintain abstinence, treat co-morbid mental health problems and reduce the risk of adverse outcomes (including death).

Traditionally, withdrawal from opiates has been managed by prescribing and administering reducing doses of either the opiate of dependence (for example, diamorphine) or another opiate agonist (for example, methadone). The choice is determined partly by the doctor's judgement on the most suitable medicine for providing even cover, partly by the expressed wishes of the patient, and partly by the social and political context within which the treatment is provided. For example, diamorphine (heroin) is never prescribed as the drug for management of the withdrawal syndrome – largely because of the sense of public outrage that would ensue and certain national prohibitions and restrictions.

Patients should be offered advice on aspects of lifestyle that require particular attention during opioid detoxification, including a balanced diet, adequate hydration, sleep, hygiene and regular physical exercise. You should develop a care plan in agreement with the patient: to establish and sustain a respectful and supportive relationship with the patient, to help the patient identify situations or states when he or she is vulnerable to drug misuse, and to explore alternative coping strategies, including the involvement of family and carers, so long as confidentiality is maintained. An important part of recovery from opioids is engagement with self-help groups, so you should provide the patient with information about groups such Narcotics Anonymous.

The NICE guideline (2007) recommends that methadone or buprenorphine should be offered as the first-line treatment in opioid detoxification. When deciding between these medications, healthcare professionals should take into account:

- whether the service user is receiving maintenance treatment with methadone or buprenorphine; if so, opioid detoxification should normally be started with the same medication;
- the preference of the service user.

Before you proceed further, try Activity 10.3.

Activity 10.3   *Decision-making*

Mavu is 30-year-old man who has been using illicit drugs since he dropped out of university 11 years ago. He uses a variety of street drugs including heroin. He informs you that he has been taking methadone as well as illicit drugs until 24 hours before he was admitted to hospital for depression.

- What should your admission assessment include?

An outline answer is provided at the end of the chapter.

Methadone

Case study

Doug is a 33-year-old man who spends an average of £200 a day on heroin. He is motivated to give up the habit and realises he needs help. He has tried to give up many times in the past but relapsed. After seeing his GP, he now takes methadone medication.

Methadone is a typical example of *replacement therapy*. Replacement therapy is the use of substances that are similar to, but less addictive than, the drug that has been abused. Methadone has been described as the most effective medicine currently used in detoxification (Faggiano et al., 2003) Methadone is a synthetic opiate whose action is very similar to that of heroin, except that it has a longer half-life and does not produce the same euphoric effects. Methadone is a full agonist that has an affinity for opiate receptors and, when taken orally, it is completely absorbed and stored in parts of the body, including the bones and liver. Methadone is slowly metabolised, reaches peak plasma levels within two to four hours after administration, and it has half-life range of between 13 and 50 hours.

As with alcohol, the opiate treatment starts with the detoxification stage. This is best carried out in a controlled environment, as evidence suggests that the setting in which the treatment is provided has a profound effect, with much greater adherence and completion rates being seen within specialist inpatient services compared with general psychiatric ward settings (Strang et al., 1997).

The dose of methadone is gradually increased from initial doses of around 10mg to 30mg daily. In clinical practice, it is important that doses should be increased slowly under supervision. It is not uncommon for people on methadone therapy to supplement their treatment with other illegal drugs, so you should conduct frequent urinary analysis. Doses of methadone are gradually reduced over a period of 10–28 days. Recently, it has been demonstrated that the detoxification process can effectively be managed within a shorter, ten-day withdrawal regime compared with the previously widely used 21-day regime (Strang et al., 1997).

Close monitoring of effects during the first two hours after ingestion is important because the slow methadone metabolisation may cause accumulation, which in turn may cause toxicity. Also, other drugs may interact with methadone and cause sedation and respiratory depression. There may be an increased mortality risk during the first weeks of treatment. Meta-analyses conclude that flexible, high-dose strategies are most effective (Bao et al., 2009). The recommended dose range is 60–100mg, sometimes up to 120mg daily. Methadone may be continued indefinitely as may be the case with Doug. The main reason for maintenance therapy with a replacement medication is that the monitored use of a prescribed addictive medication is preferable to the uncontrolled use of a more highly addictive street drug. For example, if Doug is maintained on methadone, he is less prone to commit crime to support his habit or contract a disease such as HIV or hepatitis (Kesley et al., 2006). Before you read further, please try Activity 10.4.

Activity 10.4   *Critical thinking*

It has been reported to you by another patient that Ravinder, a 30-year-old male who is on the fourth day of a heroin detoxification programme, has been secretly taking heroin in addition to the 120mg methadone he was prescribed.

• How would you respond to this situation?

An outline answer is provided at the end of the chapter.

Buprenorphine

Buprenorphine is a synthetic partial agonist that binds to the μ-opioid receptor. As a partial agonist, the maximum effect of buprenorphine is less than that of full agonists such as methadone. It binds to the receptor almost irreversibly and dissociation from the receptor is slow, which gives it a relatively long half-life. It will displace most other opioids from the receptor, and if buprenorphine is taken first, other opioids such as heroin will be unable to displace it, even in high doses. For these reasons, buprenorphine can precipitate withdrawal in users who have taken other opioids before buprenorphine, but buprenorphine maintenance may protect patients against overdosing with other opioids. The strong binding reduces the need for additional opioid use, but this may also cause problems in reversing the opioid effects with naltrexone or naloxone. Because it is a partial agonist (partly stimulates the opioid receptors), it alleviates withdrawal and craving.

Side effects of opiates and their management

This section deals with the most commonly experienced side effects of opiates (buprenorphine and methadone). The major hazards are respiratory depression and, to a lesser degree, systemic hypotension. Respiratory arrest, shock, cardiac arrest and death have occurred with the use of methadone. Other common side effects, especially with methadone, include constipation, dizziness, drowsiness, dry mouth, headache, increased sweating, itching, lightheadedness, nausea, vomiting and weakness. For the management of these side effects, please refer to Chapters 5 and 7. In certain instances, patients may develop a severe allergic reaction to methadone, in which case you should call the doctor straight away. Some symptoms that suggest someone is experiencing a severe allergic reaction are skin rash, hives, itching, difficulty breathing, tightness in the chest, and swelling of the mouth, face, lips or tongue.

Also, you should call the doctor straight away if you notice the following: confusion, excessive drowsiness, fainting, fast, slow or irregular heartbeat, hallucinations, loss of appetite, menstrual changes, mental or mood changes (for example, agitation, disorientation, exaggerated sense of well-being), seizures, severe or persistent dizziness or lightheadedness, shortness of breath, slow or shallow breathing, swelling of the arms, feet or legs, trouble sleeping, difficulty urinating, and unusual bruising or bleeding.

Opioid overdose management

In general, opioid poisoning may be a chronic problem, in which case the main complaint will be constipation and, at times, the patient may complain of nausea, vomiting or just loss of appetite. The patient may be sedated and craving for the next dose. In acute toxicity, the patient presents with drowsiness and this is more severe if alcohol has been ingested, or if other sedatives are involved. Respiratory depression may be apparent and other signs include hypotension, tachycardia and pinpoint pupils, but this sign may be absent if other drugs are involved. Evidence suggests that deaths from heroin overdose alone are uncommon.

Drug-related deaths from heroin usually involve other drugs too. If you suspect an opioid overdose, you should try to arouse the patient and, if you are unsuccessful, call for an ambulance straight away. You should establish a clear airway, adequate ventilation or oxygen therapy if consciousness is impaired. Give naloxone IV 0.4–2mg if the patient is in a coma or respiratory depression is present. Give intramuscularly if no vein is available. Repeat the dose if there is no response within two minutes; large doses of naloxone (4mg) may be required in a severely poisoned patient. If a patient fails to respond to large doses of naloxone, this may suggest that another CNS depressant, or brain damage, is present. You need to stay with the patient until help arrives.

Some dos and don'ts in nursing people with drug misuse problems

- Always ensure that you assess the patient's level of motivation and offer brief interventions focused on motivation to change.
- It is important that, before withdrawal treatment commences, you should come to an agreement in the way of an enforceable contract with the patient about the terms and conditions of treatment.
- You should never commence treatment before you do a thorough assessment of the level of substance misuse, symptoms experienced and how frequently, co-existing mental health problems, and family and social support. If a patient withdrawing from opioids reports current use of maintenance medication, you should confirm this with the treating doctor or dispensing pharmacy. Confirmation is usually in the form of a faxed letter or prescription.
- Always confirm the use of drugs from a patient by performing a urine test to ascertain the main drug of abuse as well as other drugs that the patient may have not reported.
- Methadone should not be given to patients taking respiratory depressants such as alcohol and benzodiazepines, because the risk of overdose is greatly increased.
- If a patient reports liver function problems, you should withhold giving methadone and report this to the doctor. Renal or hepatic dysfunction interferes with the breakdown of methadone and can result in the accumulation of methadone in the plasma, causing a possible overdose.
- You should be aware that medications used in detoxification are open to misuse and diversion and therefore you need to be vigilant during supervised consumption to limit the risk of concealment.
- For patients on methadone, an ECG should be recorded at regular intervals. Some authorities recommend an ECG prior to methadone commencement and then again after four weeks (period of stabilisation) and then at 6–12 months thereafter (Taylor et al., 2007).

What the patient needs to know

- Before starting detoxification you should provide the patient with detailed information about the treatment and its benefits and risks, including the risk of seizures for alcohol detoxification, or, if the patient is taking opiates, the risks of interaction between opiates and other respiratory depressants.
- You should routinely provide the patient with information about self-help groups to assist with recovery after detoxification.
- You should give the patient the option for relatives and carers to get involved in their care plan, but you should also respect the patient's right to confidentiality.
- You should provide information to the patient about the physical effects of drugs or alcohol.
- For patients taking opiates (methadone or buprenorphine), you should inform them that the medicine can make them feel sleepy and drinking alcohol will make them even sleepier. It will obviously affect their ability to operate machinery and drive.
- Patients must not take opiates within two weeks of taking MAOIs or if they are having an asthmatic attack.

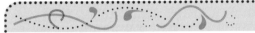

Chapter summary

The non-therapeutic use of psychoactive substances is very common and accounts for a significant proportion of the global burden of disease. The most commonly used substance is alcohol, although the use of stimulants and opiates poses a significant challenge to society because users tend to be involved in criminal acts to finance their habit. Much controversy surrounds the classification of substance misuse as a disease but, whatever one's viewpoint, there is no denying the huge personal, social, economic and health implications for the user. For this reason, people who abuse substances are entitled to the same treatment as everyone else.

Dopamine in the mesolimbic region has been implicated in addiction. A pleasurable experience is accompanied by an increase in dopamine levels in the limbic region, resulting in the reward process. Care and management of people with substance misuse disorders should always include psychosocial interventions. The treatment of substance misuse is usually in two stages, namely detoxification and maintenance or rehabilitation. In alcohol dependence, benzodiazepines are the medicines of choice during detoxification, and disulfiram, acamprosate or naltrexone are used during the maintenance phase. With regard to opiates, either methadone or buprenorphine is used both for withdrawal or maintenance. Opioid overdose can be fatal and naloxone is used to counteract the effects.

Activities: brief outline answers

Activity 10.1 Call for help from heavy drinker (pages 187–8)

The starting point is to go and see your patient as a matter of urgency. Check his level of commitment to give up drinking. The fact that he has called you is an indication that he has made some sort of commitment to giving up but may be unsure if he can. Explore ambivalence with him and offer information and treatment options. Offer detoxification, probably as an inpatient if possible. Contact his doctor and arrange for admission if needed.

Activity 10.2 Patient's drinking history (page 192)

Obtain a full history of his drinking and his reasons for drinking. Ask how it was financed as this may lead to further revelations of financial difficulties. Elicit symptoms using a scale, discuss detoxification options, and inform a doctor. Most importantly, provide support and reassurance and make sure documentation is full and complete.

Activity 10.3 Admission assessment (page 197)

You need to assess for symptoms of withdrawal, possibly using a rating scale. You need to take a history of drug usage that includes the type of drug, the quantity taken per day, and approximately how much the patient spent per day on drugs. Take a history of his methadone use, including the prescribing doctor and the dispensing pharmacy; it is vitally important to confirm the prescription or dispensing record, usually by fax. Lastly, you need to confirm which drugs the patient has been taking by undertaking a drug urine analysis.

Activity 10.4 Secret use of illicit drugs (page 199)

The supplementation of opiates with illegal drugs is not only a common problem but also hazardous. Many overdoses in people with substance misuse problems are a result of interaction between prescribed opiates and other drugs. You should therefore ask Ravinder for a urine sample to test for the presence of other drugs. If the urine test is positive for heroin or other unprescribed illegal substances, you need to inform Ravinder of this, withhold giving methadone and notify the prescriber.

Further reading

National Institute for Health and Clinical Excellence (NICE) (2010) *Alcohol Use Disorders: Physical complications.* London: NICE.

NICE produces guidelines on all types of substance misuse and their management, easily available through their website (see below).

Stahl, SM (2009) *Stahl's Essential Psychopharmacology: The prescriber's guide,* 3rd edition. Cambridge: Cambridge University Press.

A comprehensive guide to psychopharmacology that is clearly written and has good illustrations.

Taylor, D, Paton, C and Kerwin, R (2007) *The Maudsley Prescribing Guidelines,* 9th edition. London: Informa Healthcare.

This is a very useful, easy-to-understand, evidence-based prescribing and general medicines management manual.

Useful websites

www.alcoholics-anonymous.org.uk

This website provides information from people who share their experiences, strength and hope with each other that they may solve their common problem and help others to recover from alcoholism.

www.drugs.com

This very useful website has information on virtually all medicines, side effects, preparations, interactions, latest drug warnings and reported adverse effects.

www.nice.org.uk

The NICE website was launched to manage the synthesis and spread of evidence-based practice, particularly in the NHS. Its introduction has ensured that everyone working in health and social care has free access to the quality-assured, best-practice information required to inform evidence-based decision-making, quickly and easily.

www.ukna.org

This UK Narcotics Anonymous website enables people with drug problems to share their experiences and assist each other towards abstaining from drugs.

Chapter 11
Medicine interactions

Chapter aims

By the end of this chapter, you should be able to:

- understand the types and importance of medicines interactions in clinical practice;
- outline the mechanism of action of inhibitors and inducers;
- describe the role of medicines interaction and genetic variation;
- understand the role of pharmacogenetic polymorphism and ethnicity.

Introduction

> ## Case study
>
> *Jamie was 36 years old and suffered from depression; he was prescribed amitriptyline 200mg at night. Jamie also used heroin and had been struggling to abstain. He was admitted into hospital to undergo a detoxification programme, on which he was prescribed an initial dose of methadone 60mg. He was found dead early in the morning about a day after being admitted to hospital. The post-mortem report concluded that Jamie died from ventricular tachycardia, which was most likely caused by a higher than normal starting dose of methadone; however, more importantly, the interactive effects of methadone and amitriptyline played a major contributory role in the ventricular tachycardia.*

Medicine interaction is defined as the modification of the action of one medicine by another and it can be beneficial, or harmful as in Jamie's case, or it can have no significant effect. Because of the wide variety of medicines on the market and because we now live longer, there is more chance that doctors will prescribe several medicines to a patient for different ailments, which is called *polypharmacy*. Unfortunately, polypharmacy increases the risk for inadvertent adverse effects, known as *iatrogenic effects*, but this is an important preventable complication. Patients on polypharmacy and the elderly are at highest risk of medicine interactions that require hospitalisation, but many medicine interactions are not reported by patients, and Holm et al. (2010) estimated that most medicines currently used in clinical practice are effective in only 25–60 per cent of patients because of adverse interactions. Adverse events related to medicines interaction are costly and can lead to serious illness and even death, as we have seen. Clearly, medicine interaction is a problem of which you as a nurse need to be aware.

In mental health, there are many known psychotropic medicine interactions but most are not clinically significant. Much of what we know today about medicines interactions is supported by our increased understanding of molecular biology and the mechanisms involved in medicine metabolism and disposition. The main factors that determine medicine response are the blood concentration and elimination half-life of the active medicine. These are in turn determined by a number of biological and environmental factors (Dandara et al., 2001). Biological factors include the amount of medicine administered, the extent and rate of absorption, volume of distribution (determined by liver and kidney function, and body fluid balance), protein binding and localisation in tissue, biotransformation and excretion. Among the environmental factors, diet can influence medicine absorption and distribution. Smoking, concomitant uses of other non-psychotropic medications, herbal medicines and some foods can each influence metabolism. One of the most important liver enzyme systems involved in drug metabolism is known as cytochrome P450 (CYP), which we will discuss in detail later.

Medicine interactions are usually classified as pharmaceutical, pharmacodynamic or pharmacokinetic. This chapter will discuss the different types of interaction before focusing on the enzymes that are responsible for medicine metabolism. The final section of the chapter discusses the role of genetics and ethnicity in medicine interactions.

Pharmaceutical interactions

Pharmaceutical interactions occur when two or more chemically incompatible medicines are mixed outside the body before administration. An example is the incompatibility of phenobarbital with chlorpromazine or opioid analgesics when mixed in the same syringe. Pharmaceutical interaction is the least likely of the three mechanisms to cause adverse medication reaction and there are no known potentially hazardous interactions of this type with psychotropic medicines.

Pharmacodynamic interactions

> ### Case study
>
> *Mark is a 28-year-old man who has used heroin in the past and is currently being maintained on methadone. He was found unconscious one morning and all the indications were that he had taken an accidental overdose of opiates. To counteract the effects of an opiates overdose, he was given 2mg of naloxone hydrochloride, administered intravenously. After a few hours, Mark's condition improved.*

Pharmacodynamic interaction is the most common interaction encountered in clinical practice. It occurs when the medicines have their effect in the body. This type of interaction occurs when medicines compete for the same receptor or produce antagonistic effects on the same target organ or system. An antagonistic interaction is when the medicine binds to a receptor but does not activate the receptor. Many instances of antagonistic pharmacodynamic interaction are beneficial: for example, naloxone is a specific antagonist that reverses the action of morphine by competing with it for occupancy of the opioid μ-receptor, as happened to Mark in the case study. But, more often than not, pharmacodynamic interaction can be adverse. For example, antipsychotic medicines reduce the efficacy of levodopa in Parkinson's disease by blocking dopamine receptors. *Synergistic interaction* means that the effect of two medicines taken together is greater than the sum of their separate effects at the same doses. Synergic pharmacodynamic interactions can produce harmful or beneficial effects on the same target organ or system. An example is the concomitant use of an antidepressant and lithium in treatment-resistant depression. But some such interactions are harmful, as we see in the next case study.

> ### Case study
>
> *José is a 56-year-old bank worker with a history of hypertension, hypothyroidism and depression. Currently, his daily medication regimen includes levothyroxine 150mcg, and amitriptyline 200mg. He also takes other non-prescribed medicines to help him sleep, such as diphenhydramine 50mg, an antihistamine. One day he went to the pub to celebrate a friend's birthday and drank three pints of beer. Afterwards, he went home and remembered to take his antidepressants and diphenhydramine. The next day, he could not be aroused; an overdose was suspected and he was rushed to hospital.*

You must warn patients of the effects of alcohol while taking antidepressants. A good example of a harmful synergistic interaction is that of alcohol and tricyclic antidepressants (TCAs). The CNS is affected when alcohol and TCAs are taken together. In José's case, the situation was complicated by his use of a hypnotic, diphenhydramine. All three substances – antidepressants, diphenhydramine and alcohol – have the synergistic effect of depressing the CNS. Another example of a harmful synergistic interaction is that SSRIs increase the risk of gastrointestinal bleeding when taken with aspirin or other NSAIDs. This is due to the synergistic inhibition of platelet aggregation by these drugs. Before you move to the next section, try Activity 11.1.

Activity 11.1   *Critical thinking*

You are working in a mental health clinic and notice that the doctor frequently prescribes both fluoxetine and amitriptyline for depression in the same patient.

- Is there any advantage in this?
- What is the condition in depression that is likely to result from taking two anti-depressants concomitantly?

An outline answer is provided at the end of the chapter.

Pharmacokinetic interactions

In the previous section, we saw that pharmacodynamics dealt with the way a medicine affects the body. We are now going to look at pharmacokinetics, which can be defined as the effect the body has on the medicine.

Pharmacokinetics includes the study of the mechanisms of absorption and distribution of an administered medicine. It also examines the rate at which a medicine begins to work, the duration of the effect and the chemical changes of the substance in the body. Pharmacokinetics also deals with the effects and routes of excretion of the metabolites of the medicine. As we look at the different aspects of pharmacokinetics, we will examine the various possible types of drug interaction involved.

Absorption

In pharmacokinetics, absorption is the movement of a medicine into the bloodstream and involves several phases. First, the medicine needs to be introduced into the bloodstream via some *route of administration* (skin, oral, intravenous or injection) and in a specific dosage form, such as a tablet, capsule and so on. The second stage involves *dissolution*, where a medicine, say a tablet, is ingested into the stomach and then dissolves.

The rate of dissolution is a key target for controlling the duration of a medicine's effect and, as such, several dosage forms that contain the same active ingredient may be available, differing only in the rate of dissolution. For example, some medicines are prepared as slow-release, sustained-release or enteric-coated, and this all affects the dissolution rate of the medicine. If a medicine is supplied in a form that is not readily dissolved, the drug it contains may be released more gradually over time, resulting in a longer duration of action. Having a longer duration of action may improve patient adherence since the medication will not have to be taken as often. Slow-release dosage forms may also maintain the drug's blood serum concentrations within an acceptable therapeutic range over a long period. This contrasts with quick-release dosage forms, which may result in sharper peaks and troughs in serum concentrations. Before you proceed further, try Activity 11.2.

Activity 11.2   *Critical thinking*

You are the registered nurse administering medication on the ward, and you see a patient's medicine administration chart indicating lithium carbonate 800mg SR, BD (= twice daily). You have run out of high-denomination lithium carbonate tablets and decide to give four 200mg tablets. You repeat this at suppertime. Late in the evening, another nurse reports to you that the patient looks disoriented and confused and has problems with coordination.

• What do you think might be the problem with the patient?

An outline answer is provided at the end of the chapter.

Case study

Denise, a 30-year-old solicitor who suffers from bipolar disorder, was brought to A&E in a state of stupor after taking an overdose of 40 capsules of valproic acid (500mg each) several hours earlier in an apparent suicide attempt. On admission her blood pressure was 95/50; pulse was 120 and body temperature 36.5 degrees. Blood analysis revealed lactic acidosis, an indication of hypoxia. The concentration of blood serum valproic acid was 4678mmol/L (normal therapeutic range 350–690 mmol/L).

*Denise was immediately given activated charcoal by nasogastric tube and intravenous L-carnitine and sodium bicarbonate. **Haemodialysis** was then started and, by the next morning, her valproic acid blood serum levels were back to normal.*

In some situations, the way medicines are absorbed can be advantageous, as in the case of activated charcoal, which is given following an overdose of TCAs or valproic acid, as in the case study. Charcoal absorbs the antidepressant or valproic acid in the gut, thereby reducing the effects of the overdose. In some situations, however, the absorption of medicines can be adversely affected. For example, when phenothiazines such as chlorpromazine are taken with antacids, there is decreased absorption, which leads to a reduced antipsychotic effect. Once a medicine is absorbed, it will be distributed to tissues in various parts of the body.

Distribution

How efficiently a medicine is distributed between tissues is dependent on permeability between tissues, blood flow and the rate at which the tissues receive nutrients. It also depends on the ability of the medicine to bind to plasma proteins and tissue. Medicines are easily distributed in organs that receive high levels of blood and nutrients (are highly perfused), such as the liver, heart or kidneys. By contrast, organs or tissues that receive low levels of nutrients, such as muscle, fat and peripheral organs, have poor medicine distribution.

The most frequently recognised mechanism of distribution-related medicine interaction is *altered protein binding*. Many psychotropic medicines are bound to plasma proteins, but it is the free, non-protein-bound, portion of the medicine that undergoes metabolism. If there is reduced protein binding of the medicine, this increases the free medicine fraction, therefore increasing the effect of the medicine (see Figure 11.1). Medicines that are highly protein-bound, such as phenytoin, are most prone to interactions mediated by this mechanism. For example, diazepam displaces phenytoin from plasma proteins, resulting in an increased plasma concentration of free phenytoin and an increased risk of adverse effects. Before you move on, try Activity 11.3.

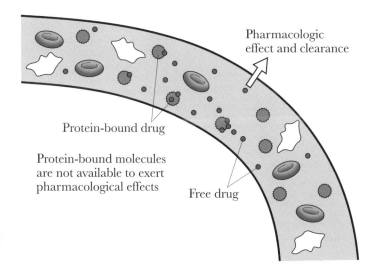

Figure 11.1: How binding to proteins affects drug interactions

---

Activity 11.3   *Decision-making*

Errol is a 54-year-old man who suffers from diabetes, hypertension and bipolar disorder. He is currently taking metformin 500mg twice a day, propranolol 40mg and his antipsychotic medication olanzapine 20mg nocte (= at night).

- How would you ensure Errol is safe from the effects of drug interaction?

An outline answer is provided at the end of the chapter.

Metabolism

In pharmacokinetics, metabolism is the chemical process that transforms a drug into another chemical. The rate of the metabolic reaction is controlled by enzymes. Enzymes are proteins found in both animals and plants, which act as organic catalysts; they help chemical reactions to proceed quickly and efficiently. Whether a medicine has a pharmacological (beneficial) or toxicological (harmful) effect largely depends on its metabolism and therefore on enzymes. Most psychotropic medicines are attracted to the fatty part of a cell membrane (that is, they are *lipophilic*), which allows them to cross membrane barriers to reach their target receptors. If the metabolites of the medicine are to be eliminated from the body, they have to be chemically transformed to more water-soluble products so that they can be excreted. This chemical process is called *biotransformation* and, if it fails, the drug can accumulate in the body, leading to the intensification of adverse effects that may be fatal.

Medicine biotransformation is controlled by enzymes called the *cytochrome P450* (CYP) enzymes, which we will discuss in more detail in the next section. The majority of these enzymes are found in the liver, the main organ involved in toxin removal from the body. A small number is also found in the small intestine. The production of CYP enzymes is controlled by a person's genes (one gene–one enzyme) and mutation in a gene gives rise to different versions of a CYP enzyme. This variation is called pharmacogenetic *polymorphism* (literally, 'many forms') and it partly explains why medicine response varies between people.

This variation of medication response and metabolism divides the population into at least three types. The first group is those people with a form of the gene (allele) that is not working or is missing. These people are called *poor metabolisers*. Poor metabolisers biotransform medicines more slowly than average, resulting in higher blood serum levels of the medicine. In practice, they require lower doses of medicine to achieve a therapeutic effect and they are prone to adverse side effects. The second group is those with an allele that is functioning normally, and they are called *extensive metabolisers*. Extensive metabolisers are able to biotransform a medicine at a normal and expected rate and therefore, in practice, require the recommended dose of medicine. The third group have an allele that is very fast at metabolising a medicine and they are called *ultra-extensive metabolisers*. These people biotransform medicines at a much higher rate than most people and, in practice, will need a higher medicine dose to achieve therapeutic effect.

The cytochrome p450 enzymes

There are as many as 50 individual CYP enzymes in humans, but many of these play a minor role in medicine metabolism. Six enzymes are responsible for more than 90 per cent of human medicine metabolism: 1A2, 3A4, 2C9, 2C19, 2D6 and 2E1. The enzymes themselves are denoted by the CYP, followed by the numeral, which denotes the enzyme family. The numeral is then followed by a capital letter that denotes a subfamily and the last numeral denotes the individual gene. Thus:

2 = family
D = subfamily
6 = individual gene.

A CYP enzyme metabolises a medicine to a compound that is readily excreted from the body. The medicine binds to the enzyme's active site and departs as a changed molecule called the metabolite. An *inhibitor* is a chemical or substance that stops or slows down the enzyme's rate of metabolising the medicine. In other words, an inhibitor stops or slows down biotransforma-tion. Some medicines act as inhibitors to the metabolism of other medicines. For example, fluvoxamine inhibits the biotransformation of olanzapine, clozapine and zotepine, if these antipsychotics are being metabolised via the CYP1A2 enzyme. In other words, when fluvoxamine is administered concomitantly with olanzapine or clozapine, it increases the blood serum level of these antipsychotics by slowing down the catalytic effect of the CYP1A2 enzyme. In the case of clozapine, the blood serum levels may be sufficiently elevated to cause seizures. In practice, the therapeutic dose of clozapine may need to be lowered if it is concomitantly administered with fluvoxamine. Clozapine and olanzapine are also catalysed by the CYP2D6 enzyme and several antidepressants are inhibitors of this enzyme; therefore, in theory, these antidepressants can cause elevation of blood serum levels of clozapine and olanzapine.

Case study

Christine, a 46-year-old woman who suffers from bipolar disorder and epilepsy, was admitted to a general ward following an infection. Before admission to hospital, she was adequately maintained on sodium valproate 800mg a day. To control the infection, she was prescribed the antibiotic ertapenem, but 21 days later she had an epileptic seizure. Her blood serum level for valproic acid was well below therapeutic levels. Ertapenem was discontinued in favour of a different class of antibiotic. After 14 days, Christine's valproic acid levels increased and were within therapeutic levels.

Alternatively, an *inducer* allows the rapid metabolism of a medicine by allowing the enzyme to act more rapidly. For example, the CYP3A4 enzyme catalyses the metabolism of several anti-psychotics, such as clozapine, quetiapine and aripiprazole, but this enzyme can be induced by carbamazepine. Concomitant administration of carbamazepine with any of these antipsychotics will lead to reduced blood serum levels of the antipsychotic, in turn leading to loss of efficacy of the antipsychotic. In practice, higher than normal doses of the above antipsychotics should be given to achieve efficacy if carbamazepine is concomitantly administered. So you need to explain to the patient the possibility of reduced efficacy due interaction.

Christine's epilepsy was stable on a dose of sodium valproate 800mg, but her blood serum levels of valproic acid were reduced substantially after she started taking the antibiotic ertapenem. The ertapenem acted as an inducer in this respect, speeding up the breakdown of valproic acid. Had the interaction between sodium valproate and ertapenem been checked prior to administration, this could have prevented Christine suffering an epileptic seizure. It is therefore important to check medicines interaction in the BNF or the internet. If you have any serious concerns, you should let the prescriber know without delay.

An important inducer of olanzapine is smoking. Smoking is an inducer of the CYP1A2 enzyme, which catalyses the metabolism of antipsychotics such as olanzapine. In this regard, doses of olanzapine may need to be increased in those who smoke. You need to inform patients of the effects of smoking on certain types of antipsychotics.

Another important area of pharamacokinetic medicine interaction is excretion, and it is that we will look at next.

Excretion

Most clinically significant medicine interactions involving excretion relate to the kidneys; the most important of these in psychiatric practice are interactions with lithium. Lithium is filtered by the kidney and reabsorbed by the *proximal renal tubule*. Incidentally, the proximal renal tubule is also where lithium is concomitantly reabsorbed with sodium. If there is sustained increase in sodium excretion, such as that produced by **thiazide** diuretics, this promotes a compensatory reabsorption of sodium by the proximal renal tubule. Lithium reabsorption is similarly enhanced. Because lithium has a narrow therapeutic window, this can increase the plasma lithium concentration to potentially toxic levels. It is therefore vital that thiazide diuretics should be avoided for any patient taking lithium.

As we have seen, genetic variations influence medicine interactions, so it follows that racial or ethnic variations between people can affect medication efficacy and side-effects profiles. A patient may prefer a particular medicine over another because that drug has been very effective for a friend, but it does not follow that the same drug will be as effective for themselves, as demonstrated by the next case study.

The importance of ethnicity in medicine interactions

Case study

Ming is a 28-year-old man of Chinese descent and he suffers from schizophrenia. For some time, he has been treated with olanzapine, but has continually complained that this drug is not effective. Also, he forgets to take his medication some evenings and has therefore asked if he could be prescribed a depot injection. In particular, he has asked for Haldol decanoate injection because his friend Jack is on this. Jack was extremely happy with Haldol and was apparently suffering no ill effects from the drug. Ming's doctor explained to him about differences in drug metabolism in different ethnic groups and added that there was a high probability that Ming would develop sexual side effects, as Haldol has been consistently associated with high prolactin levels in people of Chinese ethnicity. Having considered the doctor's explanation, Ming decided against Haldol and asked to explore other options.

Most psychiatric medications are developed and tested in North America and Western Europe. During development, these medicines tend to be tested on predominantly young, white patients. In addition, research conducted mainly in the West is extrapolated to all other parts of the world and differences in treatment response from divergent ethnic and cultural backgrounds have often been minimised or assumed to be negligible. This has led to treatment decisions that inadvertently result in suboptimal patient care. Lin et al. (1993) have argued that, unfortunately, this had led to limited treatment success and questionable acceptance in many non-Western cultures since, in any individual's response to pharmacological agents, cultural, racial and genetic factors are important.

From a genetic perspective, unique patterns exist in distinct ethnic groups, determining how the medicines are metabolised in the body and how the putative targets of medicines, such as neurotransmitter receptors, interact with the medicine. In addition, the expressions of these genes are often significantly modified by a large number of environmental factors, including diet and exposure to various substances such as tobacco, alcohol and herbal preparations. You need to inform patients of the role that environmental factors such as diet play in drug metabolism. It is therefore important for you to know if your patient is taking other herbal medicines that might interact with a prescribed medicine. If you ignore these culturally based environmental factors, the patient may not adhere to treatment fully and this may lead to treatment failure.

You should also be aware that, although there are shared biological and cultural characteristics in different ethnic groups, there is often a great danger of oversimplifying or over-interpreting results based on studies conducted in a particular group. For example, while people of Chinese ethnic backgrounds share similar cultural roots, northern and southern Chinese may diverge significantly in their genetic make-up as well as in aspects of their lifestyles, which might impact significantly on medicine responses (Chen et al., 2008). Similarly, although Africans show a unique genetic variation as a group in medicines metabolism, they also show wide inter- and intra-ethnic variations in this respect (Masimirembwa and Hasler, 1997). Therefore, during your discussion with the patient about medication, you should take these factors into account and advise patients accordingly. For example, in the above case study, the doctor rightly informed Ming about the high risk of sexual side effects. This allowed Ming to make an informed decision about his medication.

Differences in medicine responses across ethnic minority groups

There is strong evidence that convincingly confirms significant cross-ethnic medicine response variations in practically all types of medications, especially with regard to psychotropics. For example, a series of studies demonstrated that, compared to their Caucasian counterparts, Chinese patients are often successfully treated with lower dosages of haloperidol and other antipsychotic medications in inpatient settings (Chen et al., 2008). When given comparable doses of medication, Chinese schizophrenic patients and Chinese normal volunteers exhibited plasma haloperidol concentrations that were approximately 50 per cent greater than their Caucasian counterparts (Lin et al., 1988). At the same time, the study also showed a greater prolactin response to haloperidol in Chinese people than in Caucasians. These studies, among many others, suggest that both pharmacokinetic and pharmacodynamic mechanisms are responsible for observations of South East Asians requiring lower doses of antipsychotics for similar therapeutic responses. This has important clinical implications for you as a nurse, because of the need to monitor clinical responses and adverse medicine reactions from ethnic populations. In the case study above, it would also be important to inform Ming that, should he be on Haldol, he will be at an increased risk of developing EPS. Now we need to turn our attention to the role of ethnicity in medicine responses and specific types of psychotropics.

Antipsychotics

From a prescribing perspective, there is pronounced racial variation in the medicines management of schizophrenia, as reported by several authors (e.g. Mallinger et al., 2006). Chaudhry et al. (2008) have argued that this disparity may contribute to increased rates of adverse effects, lower rates of adherence and more frequent A&E visits and psychiatric hospitalisations, a finding supported by Herbeck et al. (2004), among others. With respect to clozapine and olanzapine, black patients are significantly more likely to be concomitantly prescribed other regular antipsychotics (Taylor *et al.* 2004).

Chinese and Hispanic patients have been found to need lower doses of antipsychotics to attain similar treatment responses (Chaudhry et al., 2008) and they are more sensitive to EPS (Binder and Levy, 1981). With respect to movement disorders, Oriental and Hispanic patients have significantly higher proportions of movement disorders compared to Caucasians, despite the use of lower therapeutic doses (Strickland et al., 1997). Overall, Orientals seem to have a lower threshold for both therapeutic and adverse effects with antipsychotic medication than Caucasians (Bond, 1991).

In the UK, clozapine is used much less among African-Caribbean patients than other ethnic minorities (Mallinger and Lamberti, 2006). Lower normal ranges for WBC counts in these patients (benign ethnic neutropenia) may partly explain this discrepancy and this has also been observed in Middle-Eastern ethnic groups. Ashkenazi Jews also appear to have an increased susceptibility to clozapine-induced agranulocytosis (Whiskey and Taylor, 2007).

There is a high prevalence of type 2 diabetes in South Asian and African-Caribbean populations. All atypical antipsychotic medicines can induce diabetes, but medicines such as olanzapine and clozapine have been known to induce diabetes more often than other medicines. As ethnic minority patients, including Asians, Hispanics and African-Americans are already predisposed to develop diabetes, antipsychotics increase the risk further. Such a situation poses a problem in treating ethnic minority psychiatric patients. Ethnic-based responses to antipsychotic medication are also observed with antidepressant medication. Before you move to the next section, try Activity 11.4.

Activity 11.4   *Critical thinking*

Dolores is 24-year-old black woman on your ward who suffers from bipolar disorder. Currently she is suffering from an acute episode of mania and is very restless and irritable; she has flights of ideas and is interfering with other patients, and several have lodged complaints about her manner. Attempts to divert her using psychological means of management have largely been unsuccessful. She is, however, agreeable to take medication to help her to 'slow down'. A doctor asks for your opinion of what medication to give Dolores.

* What will your response be, and why?

An outline answer is provided at the end of the chapter.

Antidepressants

As with antipsychotic medication, some key differences across ethnic groups have been reported in antidepressants in terms of the prescription, treatment responses and side-effects profiles. For example, early studies have reported that Caucasians appear to have lower plasma levels of TCAs and attain plasma peaks later when compared with Asians from the Indian subcontinent (Rudorfer et al., 1984*)*. These differences have been attributed to a greater incidence of slow pharmacokinetics among Asians compared with Caucasians. Also, another study found that lower therapeutic doses of TCAs and lithium are required in Asian populations (Okuma, 1981). Other findings that support interethnic variability in antidepressant treatment are that lower doses of antidepressants are required for Hispanic women compared to Caucasians (Sramek and Pi, 1996), and lower doses of TCAs are needed for black patients to attain similar treatment responses to those of Caucasians (Varner et al., 1998). Overall, current available evidence supports the use of lower doses of antidepressants in people of Asian origin. This is because they metabolise antidepressants at a slower rate than Caucasians. Clearly, conclusions can be drawn from these findings that dosages of antidepressants should be carefully individualised over a prolonged period.

With respect to other psychotropics, a study that investigated the use of lithium in Iran concluded that Iranians should be treated with lower doses compared to Europeans and North Americans (Hashemi and Movahedian, 2006). A different study that examined the use of lithium in African-American patients found that those with bipolar disorder were more susceptible to lithium side effects than Caucasian North Americans (Strickland et al., 1995). Another finding supporting ethnic variability in the use of psychotropic medications showed more pronounced mental and psychomotor depression in Oriental people compared to Caucasians after repeated use of diazepam (Chaudhry et al., 2008).

Overall, in spite of the ongoing debate on whether ethnicity is an important factor in psychopharmacology, it is clear that, if ethnicity is defined as shared genetic and cultural or environmental background, it is indeed an important influence on psychotropic medicine responses and interactions.

Chapter summary

Medicine interaction has become an important topic in medicines management and there are at least three types of interaction: pharmaceutical, pharmacodynamic and pharmacokinetic. Pharmaceutical interaction is where two incompatible medicines are mixed before they are ingested by the patient and is the least harmful of all medicine interactions. Pharmacodynamic interaction can be defined as what the medicine does to the body and, if two medicines that essentially work on the same receptor are given to a patient, this can give rise to synergistic effects. Pharmacokinetic interaction can be defined as what the body does to the medicine. Pharmacokinetic processes can be divided into at least four phases that include absorption, distribution, metabolism and excretion. Metabolism plays a crucial role in pharmacokinetic medicine interactions and this involves cytochrome P450 enzymes. There are approximately six main CYP enzymes that are responsible for catalysing the metabolism of most medicines. The metabolism of medicines differs across ethnic and racial lines, but there is also intra-ethnic variation that has a genetic base.

Activities: brief outline answers

Activity 11.1 Fluoxetine and amitriptyline (page 207)

- The answer is no, as polypharmacy is more likely to result in medicine interactions.
- The answer is serotonin syndrome, because of a synergistic reaction.

Activity 11.2 Lithium carbonate error (page 208)

Sustained-release (SR), sustained-action (SA), extended-release (ER, XR or XL), time-release or timed-release (TR), controlled-release (CR), modified release (MR) or continuous-release (CR) systems are used in tablets that dissolve slowly and are to be released into the bloodstream over a longer time. The advantages of SR tablets are that they can be taken less frequently than instant-release formulations of the same medicine and they keep steadier levels of the medicine in the bloodstream. Ingestion of the quick-release form of lithium carbonate (200mg) is likely to result in higher blood serum levels of the medicine. Hence, the patient is likely to be experiencing severe side effects. The medicine has not been administered correctly following prescribed instructions; this will be classed as a drug error and you will need to follow drug error procedures.

Activity 11.3 Polypharmacy risk (page 209)

Although Errol is hypertensive, he is also at risk of the effects of a drug interaction. Olanzapine may potentiate the hypotensive effect of propranolol and this may lead to Errol to develop orthostatic hypotension and **syncope**. Errol should be advised to avoid rising abruptly from a sitting or recumbent position and to notify the nurse if he experiences dizziness or lightheadedness. You should also advise him to avoid driving or operating hazardous machinery until he knows how the medications affect him.

Activity 11.4 Ethnic variation risk (page 214)

Dolores is likely to experience EPS from even relatively low doses of antipsychotic, because current evidence suggests that people from black ethnic backgrounds are prone to these symptoms even on low doses. Therefore, she might benefit more from sedatives such as benzodiazepines (e.g. diazepam or lorazepam). If the doctor decides to prescribe antipsychotics, you should explain the likely side effects to Dolores and you need to manage these side effects aggressively.

Further reading

Baxter, K (ed.) (2011) *Stockley's Drug Interactions Pocket Companion*. London: Pharmaceutical Press.

This pocket-sized book on drug interactions is easy to carry around in clinical areas.

Brolsen, K and Naranjo, CA (2001) Review of pharmacokinetic and pharmacodynamic interaction studies with citalopram. *European Neuropsychopharmacology*, 11(4): 275–83.

This is a detailed review of studies that have investigated the interactions of citalopram.

Stargrove, BM, Treasure, J and McKee, DL (2008) *Herb, Nutrient, and Drug Interactions: Clinical implications and therapeutic strategies*. St Louis, MO: Mosby.

This is a very good book that gives information of not only drug, but also food–drug interactions.

Useful websites

www.medscape.com/druginfo/druginterchecker

This very useful website allows you to enter two or more drug names, including herbal medicines, to check interactions between them. It is user-friendly and gives very detailed information.

Chapter 12
The multidisciplinary team and medicines administration

> **Chapter aims**
>
> By the end of this chapter, you should be able to:
>
> - understand interprofessional team roles, especially those of prescribers, dispensers and administrators of medicines;
> - outline the Five Rights (5Rs) of medicines administration;
> - describe medicines administration via the oral, sublingual, rectal, eye and ear routes, and intramuscular and subcutaneous injection procedures;
> - recognise common errors encountered in prescribing, dispensing and administering medicines.

Introduction

Prescribed medicines are the main intervention for the prevention and treatment of mental ill-health. Therefore, it is important that medicine is appropriately prescribed and that patients continue to get the most from medicines after taking them. Nurses can help patients get the optimum benefit from medicines through the medicines management framework.

Medicines management is one of the most complex parts of a patient's care delivery and it is not unusual for many different health professionals, departments, facilities and processes to be involved. It is clear that, without full coordination of care between the prescriber who orders the medicine, the pharmacy that dispenses the medicine and the nurse who administers it, the risk of potentially harmful medication errors increases. A good starting point in minimising these errors is for you to understand the roles of the prescriber, dispenser and administrator of medicines. This chapter will discuss the roles of each profession involved in the medication process before focusing on the administration of medicines in different formulations. First, let us look briefly at the dynamic nature of medicines management.

The changing nature of medicines management

The traditional model of medicines management suggests that this process consists of a series of stages:

1. prescribing (ordering a given medicine and dose);
2. dispensing (supplying medicines to individuals or to hospital wards);
3. preparation (preparing a dose of medicine for administration);
4. administration (administering the dose of medicine by the appropriate route and method);
5. monitoring (checking the administration and effect of a medicine).

In the traditional model, doctors prescribed, pharmacists dispensed and nurses administered medication. Now the picture is more complex. Many professionals are involved at every stage of the medication process, and medication safety has become a multiprofessional concern.

The role of the prescriber

Traditionally, the role of prescribing medication has been entrusted to doctors. Access to POMs has until recently been dependent on the written order of a doctor or dental practitioner. Doctors are eligible to prescribe all items contained within the *British National Formulary* (BNF). Recent legislation on prescribing allows other non-medical professionals, such as nurses and pharmacists, to prescribe medication. The prescriber is responsible for making a diagnosis before prescribing a medicine.

Nurses, including mental health nurses, who have completed a course in prescribing are permitted to prescribe medicines. Mental health nurses are expected to have a suitable level of background knowledge of clinical psychopharmacology and therapeutics in order to benefit fully from the training. In addition, prescribers are required to train in the following areas:

*   legislation (see Chapter 2);
*   professional role and accountability;
*   prescribing principles and procedures;
*   economic aspects.

It is generally accepted that good prescribing is based on a number of basic principles and, in 1999, the National Prescribing Centre developed a seven-step pyramid model (NPC, 1999, p2), shown in Figure 12.1.

The NPC recommends that each step should be carefully considered before moving up to the next. All treatment options should be considered, including the option not to prescribe medication. If a decision to prescribe is taken, the product or medicine that is effective, appropriate, safe and cost-effective for the patient should be prescribed. As far as possible, the patient should be encouraged to participate in the decision-making process. The prescriber should also undertake a regular review of the medication prescribed and this normally involves the prescriber meeting with the patient to evaluate treatment progress in terms of safety, acceptability and effectiveness. Once medication is prescribed, it should be dispensed and this generally involves the pharmacist. But before you proceed further, try Activity 12.1.

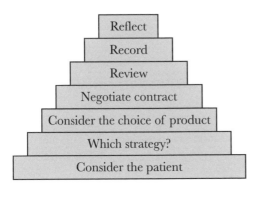

Figure 12.1: The seven-step pyramid prescribing model

Activity 12.1   *Team working*

Arrange to talk to a doctor on your team about his or her role as a prescriber. In particular, find out about the challenges of medication prescribing.

As this is an individual activity, there is no outline answer at the end of the chapter.

The role of the pharmacist

The role of the pharmacist in medication management is to promote and support the safe, effective and responsible use of medicines. The focus of a pharmacist's role is the medication needs of the patient. Recently, these patient-focused activities have evolved into the concept of *pharmaceutical care*, which can be defined as *the responsible provision of medicines with the aim of achieving desired treatment outcomes that enhance a patient's quality of life* (Hepler and Strand, 1990). In pharmaceutical care, pharmacists are directly accountable to patients for the outcomes of medicine therapies. In recent years, the role of the pharmacist has shifted from a focus on the preparation and supply of medicines to a focus on the sharing of pharmaceutical expertise and knowledge with doctors, nurses and patients. Developments in pharmaceutical care are occurring in both the hospital and in the community.

Pharmacy practice in the community

In the community, pharmacists help patients gain the maximum benefit from their medication, and are involved in dispensing and providing information and support to patients. In the management of long-term conditions, including many mental health conditions, pharmacists not only supply the medicines to patients, but are increasingly involved in the development of locally agreed shared care protocols that ensure patients use prescribed medicines to the best advantage to improve treatment outcomes.

Case study

Richard is a 26-year-old man who has been prescribed methadone replacement therapy by his doctor. He collected his medicine from his local community pharmacy. Before dispensing and administering the medicine, Satish, the pharmacist, spent some time with Richard finding out more details about his lifestyle. In particular, he asked Richard whether he felt that the dosage of methadone he was taking was sufficient. During the discussion, Satish was able to establish that Richard was still at risk of using illicit medicines while on methadone therapy. Satish explained to Richard the possible risks of taking these medicines in tandem with methadone.

In the management of common ailments such as allergies or flu, pharmacists play a vital role in supporting responsible self-medication by giving people advice and reassurance. They also supply non-prescription medicines when appropriate and refer people to other healthcare professionals where necessary.

In the promotion and support of healthy lifestyles, pharmacists help people to maintain good health by providing health screening, advice on healthy living and other services. Pharmacists are now involved in a range of such services, including blood pressure measurement, testing body fluids, cholesterol testing, pregnancy testing, smoking cessation advice and diabetes guidance. In the community, the pharmacist can, in special cases, supply POMs without a prescription on the request of a doctor or individual patient. Finally, pharmacists contribute their expert knowledge of medicines and their use for the benefit of other healthcare workers, including both doctors and nurses.

Pharmacy practice in the hospital setting

A hospital pharmacist's role has become more patient-focused, with emphasis placed on the provision of the medicines needed by inpatients. Many hospital-based pharmacists supply medicines for outpatients, together with advice and information about their use. Individual pharmacists now specialise in such areas as medicines information, formulary development and clinical trials. One of the most important developments of hospital pharmacy has been the shift in the location from within the confines of the pharmacy to the ward or clinic setting. In many places, pharmacists visit wards to check prescription sheets and to initiate supply, so as to avoid the need for prescriptions having to be sent to the pharmacy, and medicines not being available at all times on the ward. Pharmacists have become more involved on the wards, advising doctors on what might be prescribed and helping nurses with problems in medicine administration. The 'ward pharmacist', as in the case of the community pharmacist, has evolved into a more patient-orientated 'clinical pharmacist'. By visiting the ward, the pharmacist is able to obtain detailed information on the medicines prescribed for each patient and contribute in areas such as the interpretation of prescriptions, checking dosage levels and monitoring prescriptions for possible medicine interactions. By working at a ward level, the pharmacist has more access to information on a patient's clinical condition than would be the case if she or he was working solely in the pharmacy. Also, with respect to dispensing, they have to ensure that medicinal products are properly labelled.

The labelling of medicinal products

The Medicines Act 1968 stipulates that medicines should be labelled and that the label must be clear, legible and comprehensible. It further orders that the information on the label includes the name of the patient, the name of the medicine (usually its generic, rather than brand name), the preparation (e.g. syrup, tablets or capsules), the strength of the medicine, the quantity, storage instructions if applicable, route of administration, expiry date, any special warnings about the product, batch reference number and instructions for use. After medicines have been dispensed, they have to be transported and stored in a safe place. Before you go any further, try Activity 12.2.

Activity 12.2   *Reflection*

Consider, and then make a list of things that could go wrong if a medicine label is not clear.

An outline answer is provided at the end of the chapter.

Storage of medicines in hospital setting

Once medicines are ordered and transported to the ward, they should be stored in a secure locked cupboard. Separate locked cupboards should be used for clinical reagents, external medicines, internal medicines, disinfectants and antiseptics. In addition, a refrigerator with a lock is required and, within this, oral preparations should be stored separately from injections. In the case of CDs, they should be stored in a cupboard that is solely reserved for this purpose. This cupboard should be secured to the wall and, ideally, fitted with a red warning light to identify when the door is open. These cupboards may be separate from others or inside other locked medicines cupboards used to store internal medicines. The lock must not be common to any other lock in the hospital. CDs must be stored and records kept according to local policy. Now we need to turn our attention to the role of the nurse in medicines management.

The role of the nurse in medicines management

The role of the nurse in medicines management can be divided into the following areas, according to Luker and Wolfson (1999):

- to administer medicines to patients;
- to report any side effects and take action where appropriate;
- to give advice to the patient about medication and possible side effects;
- to promote patient adherence to medication;
- to provide alternative or supplementary care to medicines therapy;
- to adhere to procedures for the control of pharmaceutical products.

Your role as a nurse is more than just performing tasks mechanically; you are required to exercise professional judgement and apply your knowledge, skills and commitment. You must always be aware of the potential pitfalls of medicines administration and are therefore required to act in a way that promotes and safeguards the well-being of the patient at all times. For this reason, you are personally accountable for your own practice, and this applies to nurses in all fields of practice (see Chapter 2). As you are accountable for your actions, it is important that you acquire practical skills supported by sound knowledge, because, no matter how careful or competent the prescriber or the dispensing pharmacist, there may be adverse consequences if you are not sufficiently prepared to administer medicines efficiently.

If you are to advise patients and carry out the safe administration of medicines, you will need a good understanding of basic psychopharmacology (see Chapters 5 to 11). You need to understand prescribing, ordering and storage procedures, dosage levels and routes or methods of administration, and you will need to consult employer policies for detailed guidance. In addition to this, you need to know the mode of action of the medication, recognise side effects and signs of toxicity, and know how to manage cases of toxicity. You also need knowledge of the interactions between medicines, and between medicines and certain foods.

Case study

Yusuf, a young man suffering from schizophrenia, is on a flupenthixol depot injection. He approaches Brian, a registered nurse, complaining of a dry mouth. Brian knows that a dry mouth is a side effect of flupenthixol decanoate injection. Yusuf is prescribed procyclidine 5mg PRN (pro re nata = as needed)*, but, an hour after Brian administers to Yusuf, Yusuf approaches Brian saying that the medicine he has just given him does not work; if anything, it has made his problems worse.*

Although Brian correctly identified that Yusuf is experiencing side effects due to flupenthixol, the administration of procyclidine in this case is incorrect. Procyclidine is for the alleviation of EPS only. If anything, administration of procyclidine in this case is certain to make the condition worse, as Yusuf correctly identified. By understanding the basic theory behind medicines and the condition to be treated, you can act with precision and confidence in the exercise of your professional duties. If you lack a basic understanding of physiology and psychopharmacology, your understanding of how the medicines work is incomplete and your effectiveness in practice will be questionable. For example, if you do not have good knowledge of the physiology of the very young or very old, you may put people in these age groups at risk, as they are more prone to adverse reactions from medicines than others. Before you read further, try Activity 12.3.

Activity 12.3   *Critical thinking*

George is 76 years old and is suffering from depression. He has been referred by his GP to a psychiatric unit. George's condition has deteriorated since he started taking imipramine, a TCA. He is more confused and his appetite is now very poor. The Older Adult Psychiatrist who interviewed him was convinced George needed a change in medication. Therefore, he discontinued George's imipramine and prescribed citalopram for him instead.

•   Why did the doctor do this?

An outline answer is provided at the end of the chapter.

You should familiarise yourself with local policies and procedures related to medicines management. Above all, you need to have an understanding of the patient receiving the medicine. This information should include the patient's name, age and diagnosis. In addition, you should be familiar with patients' hypersensitivities, such as allergies or a history of adverse reactions to other medicines.

You will need to master a variety of skills to be able to manage medicines in a clinical setting successfully. One important skill is that of good observation. By accurately observing a patient's condition before and after taking medication, you should be able to assess whether treatment is indicated and is effective. This point is demonstrated by the next case study.

> **Case study**
>
> *Christine is 27 years old and takes diazepam 10mg three times a day for long-standing anxiety. Christine arrived on the ward from a day's home leave and, during medication administration time, she asked for her medication. The nurse noticed that Christine's speech was slurred and, more importantly, her breath smelt of alcohol. Upon further discussion with the nurse, Christine admitted that she had had a few glasses of wine while at home. The nurse informed Christine that she would not be able to administer medication to her until the effects of the alcohol wore off. The nurse further explained the role of alcohol and its interaction with medicines, and in this case with diazepam.*

Your observation should always include the patient's mental state as well as the presence or absence of side effects. If the nurse had not been alert to Christine's slurred speech and the smell of her breath, she would have administered diazepam, which interacts synergistically with alcohol; the likely consequence is depression of the respiratory system.

Another important skill you should develop is good communication. Of all the skills that are relevant in your work, no skill is more important than the ability to communicate with people effectively, and this has been discussed in detail in Chapter 3. During the early stages of treatment, you should try to elicit information such as any history of allergies, previous medicines the patient used to take, any non-prescribed medicines that the patient is taking, any barriers that the patient might be experiencing in taking medicines as instructed, or their general attitude towards medication. You should be able to communicate information to the patient, such as the name of the medicine, the dosage, the number of tablets to be taken at one time and the number of times a day, the likely duration before therapeutic benefits can be realised, possible side effects and their management. You should incorporate all this knowledge and these skills into your practice of medicines administration.

Medicines administration

The NPSA (2007) estimates that each hospital in England and Wales administers around 7,000 doses of medication a day. Clinical places of work have policies regarding medicines administration that are based on legal requirements, and codes of practice and standards of professional bodies such as the NMC. As a minimum requirement, you should be familiar with and adhere to the NMC *Standards for Medicines Management* (2008b) at all times.

The NMC emphasises that competency in administration of medicines is an integral and essential entry criterion for the Council's Professional Register and it clearly states that medication administration must not be seen as solely a mechanistic task, but as a task that requires thought and the exercise of professional judgement (NMC, 2008b). Further, the NMC expects nurses to demonstrate a broader understanding of the uses, action, doses and side effects of these medicines (NMC, 2008a). As previously suggested, if you are to practise competently, you must ensure you have the knowledge, skills and abilities required for lawful, safe and effective practice. You must *acknowledge your professional competence and only undertake practice and accept responsibilities for those activities in which you are competent* (NMC, 2008b). It is clear that medicines administration is a complex role that encompasses a number of tasks, including:

- administering medication safely and efficiently by following the 'five rights';
- assessing and monitoring the effects of medication;
- collaborating with other professions;
- monitoring adverse effects of medication and managing these.

Before you administer medicines, you should do a mental check on the five factors commonly referred to as the 'five rights' (5Rs).

- **Right patient**: In some instances patient medicines administration charts bear a patient's photo. Ensure you have positively identified the patient.
- **Right medicine**: You need to check the administration chart for the name of medicine and compare this with the medicine on hand. As many medicines have similar spellings, this needs to be checked carefully. It is often recommended that you do three checks of the medicine to be administered: first, when reaching for the package that contains the medicine; second, when opening the medicine; and, third, when returning the package to its storage area.

Scenario

A diabetic patient prescribed chlorpropamide was given chlorpromazine instead. Imagine the consequences of this error, for both the patient and the nurse.

- **Right dose**: You should compare the ordered dose to the dose on hand. At times, you may need to perform calculations to determine the correct dose (see Chapter 1). If you are at all unsure of your calculation, get someone to check it.
- **Right route**: You should check the medication record for how to administer the medicine, and also the medicine label to verify the prescribed route. This is vitally important for medicines that are to be injected.
- **Right time**: Verify the frequency of the dose, and that the time of day ordered matches the current time.

Scenario

A patient prescribed fluoxetine 40mg in the morning usually received his medication in the afternoon because he did not get up in time. Typically, his sleep pattern was disturbed and he was awake for most of the night.

You should handle all medicines in such a way that they do not come into contact with potentially contaminated objects or surfaces, including your own hands. You should not leave any medicines unattended, and patients should be observed taking the medication. This avoids the disposal, hoarding, abuse or misuse of the medication, and assures the safety of the patient.

Documentation of medication administration is an important responsibility. The patient medicines administration chart tells the story of what substances the patient has received and when. Like other healthcare records, it is also a legal document. All institutions have policies and procedures on documentation. As the administering nurse you will need to initial the record and enter the time and date next to the appropriate prescription. You may provide other information, such as the location, the severity of the ailment or the pulse rate for medicines such as digoxin. You should document patient refusals of medication and the reason, if possible, in patient notes and inform the prescriber.

You should document all medicine errors and notify the prescriber. Most institutional policies require you to file a separate form to document errors. Errors can include administering the wrong medicine, the wrong dose, at the wrong time or via the wrong route. Omissions of medication are also considered errors. If errors are not recorded, steps cannot be taken to avoid such errors in the future, so it is your responsibility to complete this process.

Administration of controlled drugs

Procedures relating to the prescribing, handling, storage and administration of CDs are usually drawn up by health authorities against the background of the legal and professional responsibilities defined by the Misuse of Drugs Act 1971 (see Chapter 2) and the Misuse of Drugs Regulations 1973 and 2001, among others. As with all medicines, CDs should be administered in line with the principles and guidelines laid down by your professional body (NMC, 2008b). For example, it is clearly stated that the preparation and administration of all CDs must be witnessed by two persons, one of whom must be a registered nurse or midwife (Standard 26). In cases where CDs are to be administered intravenously, this ought to be witnessed by two registrants (Standard 20). With the exception of the administration of intravenous CDs, a student nurse who has satisfied their mentor or ward manager of their knowledge and competence with medicines administration procedures may check CDs with a registered nurse.

Every column in the CD register must be completed without fail soon after administration, with the following details:

* date and time of administration;
* name of the patient;
* dose administered and any doses discarded;
* signature in full of the nurse administering the medicine and the signature of the witness;
* the remaining balance of stock, on return to the cupboard.

If you discover an incorrect entry, actual or suspected medicine loss, you should report this to the manager and to the pharmacy immediately.

You should not, under any circumstances, alter an error in the CD register; such an entry should be correctly rewritten. We will now turn to the different routes and techniques of administration.

Administration of oral medication

Case study

Ann had been working on an acute admission ward since she had qualified as a registered nurse 18 months before. It was handed over to her that a patient under her care had been prescribed phenobarbital, which needed to be administered. Ann administered the medicine as per the card, which stated phenobarbital 600mg BD. She dispensed ten tablets of 60mg. Although she thought giving ten tablets at a time was excessive, she never queried this or checked in the BNF. About two hours later, the patient was found lying unconscious in the bathroom with depressed respiration. The patient was immediately transferred to the nearest general hospital. The prescriber was notified of the events and a subsequent investigation revealed that the prescriber in fact meant to prescribe 60mg of phenobarbital.

Prescribers, even if they are doctors or pharmacists, are not immune to making errors that may not be immediately detected. You have a responsibility to ensure that patients under your care receive medicines that will produce the most benefits with minimum harm. Ann should have followed up on her instinct that ten tablets was not a sensible dose. If you feel that a dose or medicine is not correct, you should not give the medicine and should contact the prescriber without delay. By not administering medication until she was sure of the dose, Ann would have been acting in the best interests of the patient.

If you contact the prescriber to query a prescription, you should then use your own judgement as to whether to give the medication or not, taking into account the prescriber's experience. For example, an explanation given by a consultant psychiatrist with many years' experience might be considered more reasoned than an explanation given by a junior doctor at the end of a busy night shift. If you are still not sure, you can elicit the views of the pharmacist and consult the BNF before committing yourself to a decision. What is clear is that nurses protect patients every day by querying prescriptions that have raised concern in their minds, and the failure to query a prescription when in doubt has been a contributing factor that has put patients' lives at risk (Luker and Wolfson, 1999). In addition to ensuring that prescribed medicines and doses are appropriate, you should take practical steps to ensure safe and effective administration.

Oral medication administration procedure

The oral route is the most common route of administration of medicines. This is because, compared with injections, it is economically more viable and less time-consuming, it requires less equipment, and it is not associated with pain and anxiety.

Medications ingested will pass down the digestive tract to be absorbed from the small intestine into the hepatic portal vein, which goes to the liver. Once the medicine has been metabolised by enzymes in the liver, it enters the circulation and can have its systemic effect. Therefore, it is important for you to understand the pharmacology of the individual medicine. Also, before you start administering medicines, you will need the following:

- electronic prescription or paper prescription chart;
- medication formulary (e.g. the BNF) to check medicine details;
- the manufacturer's information (if required);
- disposable medicine tray, cups and spoon;
- medicine trolley, with the medicine and a tablet splitter/crusher;
- water;
- a pair of gloves.

You must follow the local Trust policy for administration of medications as institutions may vary. Before you start you should ensure that the treatment room doors are secure to avoid unauthorised entry. Avoid distractions and interruptions while making up and administering medications; this may involve you letting other members of staff know that you will not be able attend to other duties such as answering phone calls. Also, you should remember that, although the NMC (2008b) supports the single-checking of oral medication, within strict local policy guidelines and protocols, you should never single-check oral medicines as a student nurse. However, student nurses are involved in medicines administration procedures during practice learning opportunities. If double-checking is required, as in the case of CDs, all aspects of preparation, administration and documentation must be carried out from start to finish by both nurses. An important rule is never to administer medicines you have not checked yourself.

Stage 1

- **Read the prescription** carefully and, if there is lack of clarity in the prescription, including the date and signature of the prescriber, you should not give the medicine. You should contact the prescriber without delay. Make any preliminary checks and necessary observations (e.g. blood pressure) prior to administration.
- **Check the prescription chart** to ensure the right patient receives the right medicine. The prescription should be legible and should include:
  - the name of the patient;
  - the route of administration;
  - the approved name of the medicine;
  - the dose to be administered;
  - the frequency and time of administration and the duration of treatment;
  - any special instructions (e.g. with food or before food);
  - any medicine and food allergies, including alternative medicines.

  If you are in any doubt or feel you need clarification, you should contact the prescriber or pharmacist before giving the medicine. If it is necessary to rewrite the prescription, it is your responsibility to contact the prescriber before the medicine is given.

Stage 2

- **Select the medicine required** and check the label against the prescription; remove the medication from the box or bottle.
- **Prepare the medicine** and check again with the prescription for:
  - the name of the patient;
  - the name and form of the medicine;

- the route of administration;
- the calculation (if any);
- the measured dose;
- the correct date and time;
- the time of the last dose;
- the expiry date of the medicine.

Stage 3

Essentially, the stages above are a rigorous way of adhering to the principle of the 5Rs and, once you have satisfied yourself that you have followed them, you should offer the medicine to the patient. Once you are sure that the patient has ingested the medicine, you must initial or sign the medicine chart. If medicine has not been given to the patient, for whatever reason, this should be recorded in the nursing notes and the reasons stated. If you observe, or are informed of, any contraindications during administration of any prescribed medicine, you should contact the prescriber after first taking the advice of the pharmacist where appropriate. See also the section on the administration of controlled drugs (page 226) and the overview of legislation concerning CDs in Chapter 2. Before you read further, try Activity 12.4.

Activity 12.4   *Evidence-based research*

Spend some time identifying different types of medicines in the medicines storage cupboard. In your observation, note how medicines storage containers are designed and note aspects likely to induce administration errors.

An outline answer is provided at the end of the chapter.

Administration of injections

An injection is a parenteral route of administration (that is, it does not pass through the digestive tract).

There are several methods of injection, the most popular being intramuscular, subcutaneous and intravenous. In mental health practice, intramuscular (IM) injections are the most commonly administered.

Intramuscular injections

Giving injections is a regular and commonplace activity for nurses, and good injection technique can make the experience for the patient relatively painless. However, mastery of technique without developing the knowledge base from which to work can still put a patient at risk of unwanted complications.

Depending on the chemical properties of the medicine, it may either be absorbed fairly quickly or more gradually, as in the case of IM depot injections, which are probably the most commonly administered in mental health. Depot injections are pharmacological preparations that release their active compound in a consistent way over a long period. They are either solid (e.g. risperidone – Risperdal Consta) or oil-based (e.g. flupenthixol decanoate). Advantages associated with using depot injections include increased medication adherence due to reduction in the frequency of dosing, as well as more consistent blood serum concentrations of the medicine. One particular disadvantage of administering depot injections is that the medicine is not immediately reversible, since it is slowly released.

The administration of IM injections involves a complex series of considerations and decisions that include the volume of the injectate, the medication to be given, technique, site to be administered, syringe and needle size, the patient's age and the pre-existence of bleeding disorders (Malkin, 2008). The NPSA (2007) has stated that poor practices can create adverse risks for patients and healthcare workers. These can include haemorrhage in people with bleeding disorders (Plotkin et al., 2008), pain, sciatic nerve injury, injection fibrosis and infection.

Tortora and Derrickson (2008) have recommended five sites that are potentially suitable for IM injection: deltoid, dorsogluteal, ventrogluteal, vastus lateralis and rectus femoris.

Deltoid muscles are located at the lower edge of the acromial process (see Figure 12.2). They are rarely used for IM injection, particularly antipsychotic depot injections. Giving an injection at the deltoid site may be associated with discomfort and a risk of radial and branchial nerve damage. For this reason, only a maximum of one millilitre can be administered at any one time.

The *dorsogluteal* site is also known as the upper outer quadrant and is perhaps the most popular site, but it has the disadvantage that it is close to the sciatic nerve (see Figure 12.3).

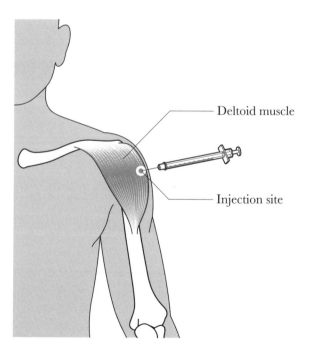

Figure 12.2: The intramuscular injection site on the deltoid muscle

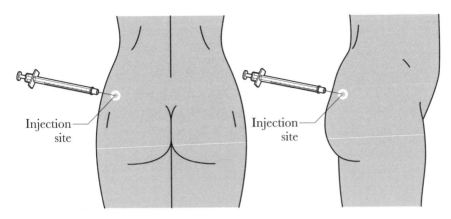

Figure 12.3: The dorsogluteal injection site

The *ventrogluteal* site is the preferred injection site for adults (see Figure 12.4). The advantages of a ventrogluteal injection are that it is reasonably free of major nerves and vascular branches. Other advantages include ease of location and a depth of muscle mass adequate enough for deep IM or Z-track injections. Injections can also be administered in numerous patient positions: supine, lateral (left or right) and on the abdomen.

The *vastus lateralis* muscle is rarely used in practice, but there are several advantages in using this method, the main one being that the muscle is normally well developed, even in children (see Figure 12.4). The injection can be given while the patient is lying flat, sitting down or on the side with the site pointing at the ceiling. A particular disadvantage of using this site is the potential for the formation of a thrombosis in the femoral artery, especially if the landmarks are not properly located.

The *rectus femoris* site is rarely used, except for infants and self-administered injections.

The volume of an injectate that can be delivered to each muscle varies; this is based on muscle size and there is little empirical evidence to support these recommendations. The maximum

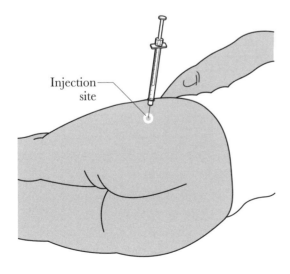

Figure 12.4: The ventrogluteal injection site

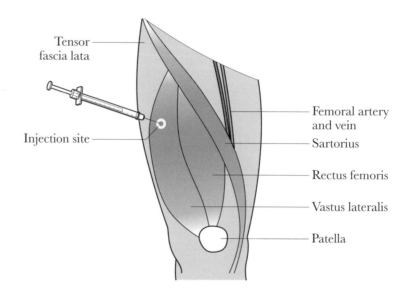

Figure 12.5: The vastus lateralis injection site

Tensor fascia lata

Injection site

Femoral artery and vein

Sartorius

Rectus femoris

Vastus lateralis

Patella

volume recommended for an adult with a large muscle is 4–5ml, and 1–2ml in a smaller muscle (Workman, 1999). There are several factors that influence patient tolerance to injections, including whether the medicine is an oil-based formulation or not, the viscosity of the medicine and the antibiotic or pH of the medicine. Therefore, at all times use your clinical judgement on what volume the individual is likely to tolerate; you can base this on the muscle size and the viscosity of the medicine. There is some evidence that smaller injected volumes help absorption and are less likely to cause a reaction (John and Stevenson, 1995). The Department of Health (DH, 2006) recommends dividing doses between two sites if the volume to be injected is greater than 3ml or 4ml. Table 12.1 gives the recommended injectate volumes for various injection sites.

Choice of needle

Most needles for injection are made of stainless steel and the diameter of the needle is indicated by the needle *gauge* (G). Needles are differentiated based on their length and diameter. The lengths of needles range from 16mm (5/8 inch) to 76mm (3 inches). In general, IM medications are given with long needles, while subcutaneous medications are given with shorter needles. The higher the needle gauge number, the smaller the needle's diameter, so a 25-gauge needle has a smaller diameter than a 19-gauge needle. Needles of the same length can have different gauge sizes.

Muscle name	Volume
Deltoid	1ml
Dorsogluteal	4ml
Ventrogluteal	2.5ml
Vastus lateralis	1ml
Rectus femoris – adults	5ml

Table 12.1: Muscle types and maximum injectate volumes

Needle gauge	Colour code
26G	Brown
25G	Orange
23G	Blue
22G	Black
21G	Green
20G	Yellow
19G	White

Table 12.2: Colour codes of needle gauges

Selection of needle gauge is made on the basis of the thickness of the medication to be given. If the medication is thick, as in the case of long-acting depot antipsychotics, a needle with a small gauge and big diameter would be chosen (e.g. 22G–19G). For each particular needle gauge, various needle lengths can be available. Table 12.2 shows the colours of various needle gauges.

In general, injections of liquid medicines, such as antibiotics, procyclidine or vitamin B_{12} are given using a 22G needle. A 22G needle is also longer (25mm in length), to enable it to reach deep into the muscle. If the medication is thicker (more viscous), as in the case of a long-acting depot injection (e.g. flupenthixol decanoate), a 20G needle may be used.

The administration of an IM injection can cause complications and potential problems include pain, anaphylaxis, and sterile and septic abscess formation if large volume injections are administered. In addition, needle phobia can develop into a long-term problem following a traumatic IM injection.

Intramuscular injection technique

The first stage of an injection technique is to let the patient know that you will be administering an injection and if they feel all right about having it. This allows time for the patient to psychologically prepare for the occasion. The second stage is to gather all the equipment you need for the injection, including the right needle, the right syringe, antiseptic pads and adhesive bandages (BandAid) on a disposable tray. Ideally, you will also need an emergency bag that contains equipment and materials to treat anaphylactic shock or cardiac arrest, in case a patient suffers either of these during or soon after an injection. At the very least, medicines to treat anaphylactic shock should be available in every room where an injection is taking place. You should bear in mind that cardiac arrest may develop as a result of anaphylactic shock, which can be caused by very small amounts of antigens. Once you have all the equipment you need, you should then follow the 5Rs (see page 225).

Before you draw the injection, you need to wash your hands as per procedure and put on disposable gloves. Draw the right amount of injectate and ensure that there are no air pockets in the injectate. You should ensure the patient's privacy and explain the injection procedure, including any potential risks. Make sure you have discussed with the patient their preferred injection site and follow the local standard operating procedure for the administration of the injection. Once the patient has consented and you have agreed on an injection site, you should clean the skin at the injection site thoroughly with an antiseptic pad (sponge with alcohol or Betadine).

You should remove the needle guard or cover by pulling it straight off, rather than using a twisting motion or a sideward motion, which may result in bending the needle. Also, avoid touching or bending the needle.

You should hold the skin around the site firmly with your free hand to reduce pain and to ensure the needle enters the correct tissue.

The needle should be inserted at a 90-degree angle, deep enough to penetrate muscle but not to touch bone. Plunge the needle firmly and quickly into the muscle to the depth of the needle with a steady straightforward motion. A quick insertion of the needle will minimise the pain for the patient.

Release the hold on the skin and move the free hand to the plunger of the syringe. Pull back the plunger until slight resistance is felt. You should check for blood entering the syringe. If blood appears in the syringe, do not administer the medication but do the following: withdraw the needle from the skin at a 90-degree angle and dispose of the needle and the syringe with its contents in a sharps box. You should then explain your actions to the patient and select another injection site. Start the injection procedure all over again. If you fail to aspirate for blood before injecting, you could administer medicine into a patient's blood vessel and this can endanger a patient's life.

When you have successfully administered the injection, you should cover the injection site by placing an adhesive bandage over the site to protect clothes from possible bloodstains and protect the injection site from infection.

After giving the injection you should observe the patient for unusual reactions, as any medication can cause anaphylaxis. You should also let the patient know that you will return to see if he or she is all right and tell the patient to let you know of any adverse reaction as soon as possible. You should sign the patient medicine chart and record the administration of the injection in the patient's notes. The information to be recorded should include the name of the medication, dose, route, muscle site, date and time. If the injection is a repeat depot antipsychotic, you should state when it is due to be given.

Subcutaneous injections

The subcutaneous route is the administration of medication into the tissue just below the skin and is commonly used in diabetes and with some vaccines. Examples of medicines given via the subcutaneous route include insulin, opioids and hormone treatments. Absorption of medication from the subcutaneous route is slower than from the IM route, and rate of absorption varies depending on the site used. Potential injection sites include the abdomen, buttocks, hips, lateral aspects of the thigh and upper outer arms. The route is most frequently used for the administration of insulin in people with type 1 diabetes mellitus. It is important that insulin is absorbed at the same rate and time every day and, ideally, at the same injection site, for example the upper arm in the morning.

Subcutaneous injection technique

The technique is similar to giving an IM injection, except you use a much shorter 25G 19mm or 27G 13mm needle. You should give the injection at a 90-degree or 45-degree angle depending on the amount of skin that can be grasped between the thumb and first finger. If you can grasp approximately 51mm (2 inches) of skin, you can give the injection at a 90-degree angle. Alternatively, if you can grasp only 25mm (1 inch), you can give the injection at a 45-degree angle. You do not need to aspirate the needle to check if a blood vessel has been punctured as this is unlikely. Wash your hands and document in the same way as for other medication.

Rectal administration

Medication can be administered via the rectal route in the form of suppositories and liquids. The rectal route is particularly useful when oral medication cannot be tolerated due to nausea, vomiting or loss of consciousness.

Before starting the procedure, you should wash your hands to reduce the risk of cross-infection and explain the procedure to the patient. You should be alert to cultural sensitivities, as people from other cultures may find rectal administration of medicines unacceptable, and you should obtain clear consent. You should wear gloves and position the patient comfortably on one side with one leg flexed. The tip of the suppository or enema can be moistened with water or a water-based lubricant (such as K-Y gel) before inserting. The rounded ended of the suppository is gently inserted into the anus and propelled forward. If possible, the patient can be asked to 'hold on' to the suppository for 5 minutes.

Sublingual administration

Sublingual (and also buccal) medications are administered to be absorbed rapidly into the bloodstream through the mucous membranes of the mouth. When a medicine comes into contact with the mucous membrane beneath the tongue (or the buccal mucosa inside the cheeks or lips), it diffuses into the profusion of connective capillaries under the epithelium and into the venous circulation. This is in contrast to oral medication, which passes through the intestines and is subject to *first-pass metabolism* in the liver before entering the general circulation.

The sublingual method of administration has advantages over oral administration in that it is more direct, and there is little medicine degradation due to first-pass metabolism from hostile stomach acid, bile or gut enzymes. Additionally, oral medication must pass through the liver where it may be chemically altered before it exerts its therapeutic effect. One disadvantage of using the sublingual method is that, if acid or caustic medicines are used long term, it can cause tooth discolouration and decay.

One commonly administered medicine using the sublingual route in mental health is buprenor-phine, which is used as replacement therapy for substance misuse. You should not administer sublingual medicines in patients with inflamed mucous membranes or open sores.

As with administration of most types of medicines, you need to wash your hands first and wear non-sterile gloves. You should then ask the patient to open the mouth with the tongue lifted. The medicine is then placed between the bottom part of the tongue and the lower gum (in buccal administration, the medicine is placed between the teeth and the cheek). You should ask the patient to keep the medicine in position until it dissolves.

Medication errors

A medication error can be defined as a failure in the treatment process that leads to, or has the potential to lead to, harm to the patient (Williams, 2007). In broad terms, they are errors in the prescribing, dispensing or administration of a medicine, irrespective of whether such errors lead to adverse consequences or not (NPSA, 2007). Medication errors can cause unnecessary pain and harm to patients and can even lead to death. In addition, they account for a substantial amount of NHS resources. In 2004, the Department of Health estimated the costs of medication-related admissions to hospitals to be in the order of £200–400 million a year. The annual cost of these avoidable admissions translates to about £359 million across the NHS in England (NPSA, 2007). The NPSA (2009) received 100 medication incident reports of death or severe harm. Most serious incidents were caused by errors in medicine administration (41 per cent) and, to a lesser extent, prescribing (32 per cent). Medication errors involving injectable medicines represented 62 per cent of all reported incidents leading to death or severe harm. The NPSA further reports that medication is the third most frequently reported incident type after patient accident and treatment/procedure. Three medication incident types – unclear/wrong dose or frequency, wrong medicine and omitted/delayed medicines – accounted for accounted for 71 per cent of fatal and serious harm. Whether they are mistakes, slips or lapses, the NPSA recognises that the majority of errors were not the result of reckless behaviour on the part of healthcare professionals, but occurred as a result of the complex nature of medicines management (NPSA, 2007, 2009). Medicine errors are the single most preventable cause of patient harm and they can occur at all stages of the medication process.

Prescribing errors

In medicines management, prescription is the first stage of the process and errors at this point can result in problems downstream. Prescribing errors are usually characterised by incorrect medicine selection for a patient, including dose, quantity, prescribing a contraindicated medicine, poor knowledge of the prescribed medicine and its recommended dose, and poor knowledge of the patient's details. Other contributing factors include illegible handwriting, inaccurate recording of medication history, confusion involving the medicine's name, inappropriate use of decimal points, and lack of a zero preceding a decimal point (e.g. 0.1). Similarly, tenfold errors in dosage have occurred as a result of the use of a trailing zero (e.g. 1.20). The use of abbreviations has led to confusion (e.g. AZT for azathioprine and zidovudine (formerly called azidothymidine), as has the use of verbal orders.

Dispensing errors

Dispensing errors can occur at any stage of the dispensing process, from the receipt of the prescription in the pharmacy to the supply of a dispensed medicine to the patient, and include the selection of the wrong strength or product. This occurs primarily with medicines that have a similar name or appearance. Lasix (frusemide) and Losec (omeprazole) are examples of proprietary names which, when handwritten, look similar. This further emphasises the need to prescribe generically (Williams, 2007). Other examples of pairs of medicines with similar names include lorazepam and lormetazepam, and amiloride and amlodipine tablets. Other potential dispensing errors include the wrong dose, the wrong medicine or the wrong patient. The use of computerised labelling has led to typing errors, which are among the leading causes of dispensing errors. Methods for reducing errors include separating medicines with a similar name or appearance, keeping disruptions in the dispensing procedure to a minimum and reducing the workload of the dispenser to a manageable level.

Administration errors

Administration errors are a result of discrepancy between the medicine received by the patient and the medicine intended by the prescriber. In other words, administration error occurs when any of the 5Rs are violated (see page 225). Administration errors have long been associated with one of the highest risk areas in nursing practice and, in most cases, involve errors of omission where the medicine has not been administered for whatever reason. Other types of errors include the administration of incorrect or expired medicines.

Contributing factors to medicine administration errors include a failure to check the patient's identity prior to administration and the storage of similar preparations in similar areas. Environmental factors such as noise, interruptions while undertaking a medicine round, and poor lighting may also contribute to these errors. The likelihood of error is also increased where more than one tablet is required to supply the correct dose, or where a calculation to determine the correct dose is undertaken. Approaches to reduce medicine administration errors should include:

- checking the patient's identity, particularly of older people with dementia;
- ensuring that dosage calculations are checked independently by another healthcare professional before the medicine is administered;
- ensuring that the prescription, medicine and patient are in the same place in order that they may be checked against one another;
- ensuring that the medication is given at the correct time;
- minimising interruptions during medicine rounds.

Clinical pharmacists are important in the safe use of medicines and, if a system exists whereby pharmacists visit the wards daily, it places them in a good position to recognise particular training needs that can be addressed (Williams, 2007).

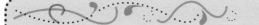

Chapter summary

The management of medicines is now a complex procedure and involves many professionals. In many cases, medicines management involves the prescriber, dispenser and administrator of the medicine. The traditional model is that the doctor prescribes, the pharmacist dispenses and the nurse administers medicines. Recent changes in medicines

continued . . .

management have changed this approach. Many professionals, including nurses, midwives, physiotherapists, dentists and psychologists can prescribe medicines after additional training. The role of the prescriber remains that of making a diagnosis, prescribing medicines and reviewing the effects. The pharmacist's role in modern medicines management is more complex; apart from dispensing medicines, they are also involved in providing expert advice on the usage of medicines to other professionals as well as patients. Pharmacists have become increasingly ward-based. In mental health, the administration of medicines requires that nurses are familiar and competent in several methods, including oral, intramuscular, subcutaneous, sublingual and rectal. Medicines management gives rise to medicines errors, some of which can be fatal, so steps to minimise errors should be put in place.

Activities: brief outline answers

Activity 12.2 Unclear labelling (page 221)

If the medicine's label is not clear, this could result is a variety of errors that include giving the medicine to the wrong person, or giving the wrong preparation, using the wrong route of administration or storing the medicines inappropriately.

Activity 12.3 TCAs and older people (page 223)

TCAs are not particularly suitable for older people because they are more prone to adverse effects such as dry mouth, constipation and cardiotoxicity.

Activity 12.4 Storage containers and drug errors (page 229)

You are likely to observe that different dosages of a particular medicine (e.g. olanzapine) have very similarly designed containers and this is a common source of error.

Further reading

Lawson, E and Hennefer, D (2010) *Medicines Management in Adult Nursing.* Exeter: Learning Matters.

O'Brien, M, Spires, A and Andrews, K (2011) *Introduction to Medicines Management in Nursing.* Exeter: Learning Matters.

These two books in the same series cover many topics that are relevant to mental health nursing.

Useful websites

www.nmc-uk.org/Nurses-and-midwives/Advice-by-topic/A/Advice/Covert-administration-of-medicines

This NMC website offers advice on the covert administration of medicines.

Glossary

Agranulocytosis: a marked decrease in the number of white blood cells called granulocytes that are responsible for fighting infection.

Ambivalence: feeling two ways about something; ambivalence is a natural phase in the process of change and must be resolved for change to occur.

Anabolic steroids: drugs that mimic the effects of the male sex hormones; they enhance protein synthesis within cells, which results in the build-up of cellular tissue, particularly muscles.

Angioedema: a swelling beneath the surface of the skin caused by a collection of fluid.

Anhedonia: loss of the ability to experience pleasure from normally pleasurable experiences.

Aplastic anaemia: a condition where bone marrow does not produce sufficient new cells to replenish blood cells. Patients with aplastic anaemia have lower counts of all three blood cell types (red and white blood cells and platelets).

Basal ganglia: a collection of nuclei found on both sides of the thalamus. It is mainly in the basal ganglia that the neurotransmitter GABA plays an important role.

Blood therapeutic drug levels: laboratory tests that look for the presence and the amount of specific drugs in the blood.

Cardiotoxicity: damage to the heart muscle, sometimes due to medications a patient is taking.

Circumstantial speech: speech in which a conversation drifts, but often comes back to the point.

Cognitive dysfunction: an unusually poor mental function, associated with confusion, forgetfulness and difficulty concentrating.

Collaborative process: chieving a desired outcome in the most efficient and effective way possible by paying much attention to how people work together in an equitable partnership.

Co-morbid substance misuse see *Dual diagnosis*

Concordance: the extent to which a patient correctly follows medical advice. It often refers to medication adherence but may also involve non-adherence to self-directed physiotherapy exercises or other courses of therapy. Both the patient and the healthcare provider affect adherence and a positive nurse–patient relationship is the most important factor.

Counter-transference: the redirection of a therapist's feelings towards a client or, more generally, a therapist's own emotional involvement with a client.

Creatine phosphokinase: an enzyme whose elevated levels in the blood are a marker for myocardial infarction (heart attack).

Cushing's syndrome: a disease caused by increased production of cortisol or by excessive use of cortisol or other steroid hormones.

Decimal: relating to a system of numbers and arithmetic based on the number ten.

Decompensation: the deterioration of a previously working structure or system. It can occur due to tiredness, stress, illness or old age. Decompensation also describes an inability to compensate for these.

Digit: any of the numbers from 0 to 9.

DNA: deoxyribonucleic acid, which is a substance present in nearly all living organisms and carries genetic information.

Dual diagnosis: also known as co-morbid substance misuse, a dual condition where a person suffers from a mental illness and a substance abuse problem. The term can be used broadly, for example depression and alcoholism, or it can be restricted to specify severe mental illness and substance misuse disorder.

Dyslipidaemia: an abnormal amount of fat, including cholesterol, in the blood. Most dyslipidaemias are hyperlipidaemias, an elevation of lipids in the blood, often due to lifestyle and diet. Prolonged elevation of insulin levels in the blood can lead to dyslipidaemia.

Ego-syntonic: a psychological term referring to behaviours, values or feelings that are in harmony with, or acceptable to, the needs and goals of one's ideal self-image.

Empirical study: a study relying on, or derived from, observation or experiment.

Exfoliative dermatitis: scaly eruption of most of the skin.

Expressed emotion: a qualitative measure of the amount of emotion displayed, typically in the family setting, usually by a family or caretakers. Theoretically, a high level of EE in the home can worsen the prognosis in patients with mental illness, or act as a potential risk factor for the development of psychiatric disease.

Extrapyramidal side effects (EPS): a group of symptoms that can occur when taking antipsychotic medications. These symptoms include akathisia, slurred speech, dystonia, slowness of movements and muscular rigidity.

Follicle-stimulating hormone (FSH): a hormone found in humans that regulates growth, pubertal development and reproductive processes of the body.

Fraction: a numerical quantity that is not a whole number, e.g. three-quarters or one-fifth.

Glial cells: supportive cells surrounding neurons in the central nervous system that do not conduct electrical impulses.

Haemodialysis: a method for removing waste products such as creatinine and urea, as well as free water, from the blood when the kidneys have failed.

Half-life: the period it takes for a medicine being metabolised to decrease by half.

Hallucinogens: drugs that cause profound distortions in a person's perceptions of reality. Under the influence of such drugs, people can see images, hear sounds and feel sensations that seem real but do not exist. An example is LSD.

Homeostasis: maintenance of a stable equilibrium in the body, especially by adjusting physiological processes.

Hyperprolactinaemia: the presence of abnormally high levels of prolactin in the blood.

Hyper-reflexia: overactive or exaggerated reflexes, such as twitching.

Hypoglycaemia: a condition that occurs when blood sugar (glucose) is too low.

Hyponatraemia: an electrolyte disturbance in which the sodium concentration in the serum is lower than normal. It is quite often a complication of other physical illness, such as vomiting or diarrhoea, where there is a loss of sodium.

Hypothyroidism: a condition in which the thyroid gland does not make enough thyroid hormone, which can result in symptoms such as increased sensitivity to cold, constipation, depression, fatigue or feeling slowed down, and heavier menstrual flow.

Idiopathic: arising spontaneously or from an unknown cause. Used to describe medical conditions where the cause is not readily apparent or understood.

Idiosyncratic response: a subjective or unusual response to a drug that is peculiar to the individual who manifests the response.

Insight: from a psychiatric perspective, this is to see ourselves as others see us.

Luteinising hormone (LH): also known as lutropin, a hormone produced by the anterior pituitary gland. It triggers the ovulation process in women. It is called the interstitial cell-stimulating hormone (ICSH) in males and is responsible for stimulating the production of testosterone.

Metabolite: a substance produced by metabolism, or by a metabolic process.

Myelin: the fatty substance that covers and protects nerves. It allows efficient conduction of action potentials down the axon. It consists of 70 per cent lipids and phospholipids and 30 per cent proteins.

Orthostatic hypotension: also known as postural hypotension, this is a form of hypotension in which the blood pressure suddenly falls when the person stands up or stretches. The decrease is most pronounced after resting. Many psychotropic medications, especially antipsychotics, cause orthostatic hypotension.

Per cent: one part in every hundred, e.g. 25 per cent is 25 out of every hundred.

Pharmacotherapy: treatment of disease with medicines.

Psychoactive: describes a chemical that crosses the blood–brain barrier and acts primarily upon the central nervous system, where it affects brain function, resulting in changes in perception, mood, consciousness, cognition and behaviour.

Psychotropic medication: medication that affects the mind, emotions and behaviour. Psychotropic medications include most medicines used to treat psychiatric symptoms.

Psychomotor arousal: unintentional and purposeless motions caused by anxiety, including pacing, wringing the hands or biting the nails.

Secondary delusions: delusions influenced by the person's background or current situation (e.g. ethnic or sexual orientation, or religious beliefs).

Sedation: an act of calming by administering certain medicines.

Steady state: a condition in the body whereby drug blood serum levels do not change over time, or in which any one change is continually balanced by another, such as the stable condition of a system in equilibrium.

Sub-therapeutic: below the dosage levels used to treat diseases.

Syncope: temporary loss of consciousness caused by low blood pressure.

Tardive dyskinesia: a movement disorder caused by long-term use of antipsychotic medications. It is characterised by uncontrolled facial movements such as protruding tongue, chewing or sucking motions and making faces.

Therapeutic alliance: within the context of psychotherapy, the collaborative relationship between therapist and client. The therapeutic alliance can have three components: an agreement between therapist and client about the goals of treatment; an agreement about the therapy tasks needed to accomplish those goals; and the emotional bond developed between therapist and client that allows the client to make therapeutic progress.

Thiazide: a diuretic medicine that increases the amount of water passed through the kidneys.

Titrating: incremental increase or decrease in drug dosage to a level that provides the optimal therapeutic effect.

Tricyclic: an antidepressant drug named after its chemical structure, which has three rings of atoms.

Trigeminal neuralgia: a nerve disorder that causes a stabbing or electric shock-like pain in parts of the face.

Validity: in research, the degree to which a study accurately reflects or assesses the specific concept that the researcher is attempting to measure.

References

Akimova, E, Lanzenberger, R and Kasper, S (2009) The serotonin-1A receptor in anxiety disorders. *Biological Psychiatry*, 66: 627–35.

American Psychiatric Association (APA) Task Force (1990) *Benzodiazepine Dependence, Toxicity, and Abuse.* Washington, DC: APA.

Anderson, A (2007) *Anxiety-Panic History: Anxiety, disorders and treatment throughout the ages.* Available online at http://anxiety-panic.com/history/h-main.htm (accessed 4 June 2011).

Anderson, IM, Ferrier, IN and Baldwin, RC et al. (2008) Evidence-based guidelines for treating depressive disorders with antidepressants: a revision of the 2000 British Association for Psychopharmacology guidelines. *Journal of Psychopharmacology*, 22: 343–96.

Areosa, SA, Sherriff, F and McShane, R (2005) Memantine for dementia. *Cochrane Database Systematic Review*, CD003154.

Ballard, C, Fossey, J and Chithramohan, R et al. (2001) Quality of care in private sector and NHS facilities for people with dementia: cross-sectional survey. *British Medical Journal*, 323: 426–7.

Bandura, A (1991) Self-efficacy mechanism in psychological activation and health promoting behaviour, in Madden, J (ed.) *Neurobiology of Learning and Affect*, New York: Raven Press, pp229–70.

Bao, YP, Liu, ZM and Epstein, DH et al. (2009) A meta-analysis of retention in methadone maintenance by dose and dosing strategy. *American Journal of Drug and Alcohol Abuse*, 35: 28–33.

Bartkó, G, Herczog, I and Zador, G (1988) Clinical symptomatology and drug compliance in schizophrenic patients. *Acta Psychiatrica Scandinavica*, 77: 74–6.

Bebbington, PE (1995) The content and context of compliance. *International Clinical Psychopharmacology*, 9(Suppl. 5): 41–50.

Becker, MH and Maiman, LA (1975) Sociobehavioral determinants of compliance with health and medical care recommendations. *Medical Care*, 13(1): 10–24.

Berghmans, R, Dickenson, D and Meulen, RT (2004) Mental capacity: in search of alternative perspectives. *Health Care Analysis*,12: 251–63.

Berk, M, Berk, L and Castle, D (2004) A collaborative approach to the treatment alliance in bipolar disorder. *Bipolar Disorder*, 6: 504–18.

Binder, RL and Levy, R (1981) Extrapyramidal reactions in Asians. *American Journal of Psychiatry*, 138: 1243–4.

Bond, DJ, Kauer-Sant'Anna, M, Lam, RW and Yatham, LN (2010) Weight gain, obesity, and metabolic indices following a first manic episode: prospective 12-month data from the Systematic Treatment Optimization Program for Early Mania (STOP-EM). *Journal of Affective Disorders*, 124: 108–17.

Bond, WS (1991) Ethnicity and psychotropic drugs. *Clinical Pharmacy*, 10: 467–70.

Borrelli, B, Riekert, KA, Weinstein, A and Rathier, L (2007) Brief motivational interviewing as a clinical strategy to promote asthma medication adherence. *Journal of Allergy and Clinical Immunology*, 120 (5): 1023–30.

Caine, ED and Polinsky, RJ (1979) Haloperidol-induced dysphoria in patients with Tourette syndrome. *American Journal of Psychiatry*, 136: 1216–17.

Carlsson, A and Lindqvist, M (1963) Effect of chlorpromazine or haloperidol on formation of 3-methoxytyramine and normetanephrine in mouse brain. *Acta Pharmacologica et Toxicologica*, 20: 140–4.

Caton, CL, Goldstein, JM, Serrano, O and Bender, R (1984) The impact of discharge planning on chronic schizophrenic patients. *Hospital and Community Psychiatry*, 35: 255–62.

Chaudhry, I, Neelam, K, Duddu, V and Husain, N (2008) Ethnicity and psychopharmacology. *Journal of Psychopharmacology*, 22: 673–80.

Chen, CH, Chen, CY and Lin, KM (2008) Ethnopsychopharmacology. *International Review of Psychiatry*, 20: 452–9.

Chessick, CA, Allen, MH and Thase, M et al. (2006) Azapirones for generalized anxiety disorder. *Cochrane Database Systematic Review*, CD006115.

Cosgrove KP (2010) Imaging receptor changes in human drug abusers. *Current Topics in Behavioural Neuroscience*, 3: 199–217.

Cunningham Owens, DG (1999) *A Guide to the Extra Pyramidal Side Effects of Antipsychotic Medicines.* Cambridge: Cambridge University Press.

Dandara, C, Masimirembwa, CM and Magimba, A et al. (2001) Genetic polymorphism of CYP2D6 and CYP2C19 in east- and southern African populations including psychiatric patients. *European Journal of Clinical Pharmacology*, 57: 11–17.

de Lima, MS, de Oliveira Soares, BG, Reisser, AA and Farrell, M (2002) Pharmacological treatment of cocaine dependence: a systematic review. *Addiction*, 97: 931–49.

Department of Health (DH) (1999) *Effective Care Coordination in Mental Health Services: Modernising the care programme approach.* London: HMSO.

Department of Health (DH) (2006) *Cardiovascular Disease and Air Pollution.* Committee on the Medical Effects of Air Pollutants. London: Department of Health.

Dorevitch, A, Aronzon, R and Zilberman, L (1993) Medication maintenance of chronic schizophrenic out-patients by a psychiatric clinical pharmacist: 10-year follow-up study. *Journal of Clinical Pharmacy and Therapeutics*, 18: 183–6.

Faggiano, F, Vigna-Taglianti, F, Versino, E and Lemma, P (2003) Methadone maintenance at different dosages for opioid dependence. *Cochrane Database Systematic Review*, CD002208.

Featherstone, RE, Kapur, S and Fletcher, PJ (2007) The amphetamine-induced sensitized state as a model of schizophrenia. *Progress in Neuro-psychopharmacology and Biological Psychiatry*, 31: 1556–71.

Frangou, S, Sachpazidis, I, Stassinakis, A and Sakas, G (2005) Telemonitoring of medication adherence in patients with schizophrenia. *Telemedicine Journal and E-health*, 11: 675–83.

Frank, AF and Gunderson, JG (1990) The role of the therapeutic alliance in the treatment of schizophrenia. Relationship to course and outcome. *Archives of General Psychiatry*, 47: 228–36.

Gabbard, GO (2005) Does psychoanalysis have a future? Yes. *Canadian Journal of Psychiatry*, 50: 741–2.

Gauthier, S, Vellas, B, Farlow, M and Burn, D (2006) Aggressive course of disease in dementia. *Alzheimers & Dementia*, 2: 210–17.

Gibb, B (2007) *The Rough Guide to the Brain.* New York: Rough Guides.

Glazer, WM, Morgenstern, H and Doucette, JT (1993) Predicting the long-term risk of tardive dyskinesia in outpatients maintained on neuroleptic medications. *Journal of Clinical Psychiatry*, 54: 133–9.

Goldberg, HL (1979) Buspirone–a new antianxiety agent not chemically related to any presently marketed drugs (proceedings). *Psychopharmacology Bulletin*, 15: 90–2.

Gonzalez-Pinto, A, Alberich, S and Barbeito, S et al. (2010) Different profile of substance abuse in relation to predominant polarity in bipolar disorder: the Vitoria long-term follow-up study. *Journal of Affective Disorders*, 124: 250–5.

Gossop, M (1990) The development of a Short Opiate Withdrawal Scale (SOWS). *Addictive Behaviour*, 15: 487–90.

Hashemi, J and Movahedian, A (2006) Lithium ratio in bipolar patients in Isfahan. *Journal of Research in Medical Sciences*, 11(4): 257–262.

Hepler, CD and Strand, LM (1990) Opportunities and responsibilities in pharmaceutical care. *American Journal of Hospital Pharmacy*, 47: 533–43.

Herbeck, DM, West, JC and Ruditis, I et al. (2004) Variations in use of second-generation antipsychotic medication by race among adult psychiatric patients. *Psychiatric Services*, 55: 677–84.

Holm (2008) Pharmacogenetics, race and global injustice. *Developing World Bioethics*, 8 (2): 82–3.

John, A and Stevenson, T (1995) A basic guide to the principles of medicine therapy. *British Journal of Nursing*, 4: 1194–8.

Johnson, JA and Bootman, JL (1995) Drug-related morbidity and mortality: a cost-of-illness model. *Archives of Internal Medicine*, 155: 1949–56.

Jukes, L and Gilchrist, M (2006) Concerns about numeracy skills of nursing students. *Nurse Education in Practice*, 6: 192–8.

Julius, RK, Novitsky, MA Jr and Dubin, WR (2009) Medication Adherence: A review of the literature and implications for clinical practice. *Journal of Psychiatric Practice*, 15 (1): 34.

Kales, A, Scharf, MB and Kales, JD (1978) Rebound insomnia: a new clinical syndrome. *Science*, 201: 1039–41.

Kaplan, HI and Saddock, BJ (1998) *Synopis of Psychiatry.* London: Lippincott Williams & Wilkins.

Kashner, TM, Rader, LE and Rodell, DE et al. (1991) Family characteristics, substance abuse, and hospitalization patterns of patients with schizophrenia. *Hospital and Community Psychiatry*, 42: 195–6.

Kesley, J (2006) *Principles of Psychopharmacology for Mental Health Professionals.* Chichester: Wiley.

Kinderman, P and Bentall, RP (1996) Self-discrepancies and persecutory delusions: evidence for a model of paranoid ideation. *Journal of Abnormal Psychology*, 105: 106–13.

Kinney, C (1999) *Coping with Schizophrenia: The significance of appraisal.* Manchester: University of Manchester.

Knapp, M, King, D, Pugner, K and Lapuerta, P (2004) Non-adherence to antipsychotic medication regimens: associations with resource use and costs. *British Journal of Psychiatry*, 184: 509–16.

Krupnick, JL, Sotsky, SM and Simmens, S et al. (1996) The role of the therapeutic alliance in psychotherapy and pharmacotherapy outcome: findings in the National Institute of Mental Health Treatment of Depression Collaborative Research Program. *Journal of Consulting and Clinical Psychology*, 64: 532–9.

Landen, M, Hogberg, P and Thase, ME (2005) Incidence of sexual side effects in refractory depression during treatment with citalopram or paroxetine. *Journal of Clinical Psychiatry*, 66: 100–6.

Lanzenberger, RR, Mitterhauser, M and Spindelegger, C et al. (2007) Reduced serotonin-1A receptor binding in social anxiety disorder. *Biological Psychiatry*, 61: 1081–9.

Lau, RR, Bernard, TM and Hartman, KA (1989) Further explorations of common-sense representations of common illnesses. *Health Psychology*, 8: 195–219.

Leventhal, H, Nerenz, DR and Steele, DF (1984) Illness representations and coping with health threats, in Baum, A and Singer, J (eds) *A Handbook of Psychology and Health.* Hillsdale, NJ: Erlbaum, pp219–52.

Lewis, F and Batey, M (1982) Clarifying autonomy and accountability in nursing services. *Journal of Nursing Administration*, 12(9): 13–18.

Lin, KM, Poland, RE, Lau, JK and Rubin, RT (1988) Haloperidol and prolactin concentrations in Asians and Caucasians. *Journal of Clinical Psychopharmacology*, 8: 195–201.

Lin, KM, Poland, RE and Nakasaki, G (eds) (1993) *Psychopharmacology and Psychobiology of Ethnicity.* Washington, DC: American Psychiatric Press.

Loffler, W, Kilian, R, Toumi, M and Angermeyer, MC (2000) Schizophrenic patients' subjective reasons for compliance and noncompliance with neuroleptic treatment. *Pharmacopsychiatry*, 36: 105–12.

Lomas, C (2009) Mental health nurses 'under-report' drug errors. *Nursing Times*, 12 May. Available online at www.nursingtimes.net (accessed 22 April 2011).

Lopez-Munoz, F and Alamo, C (2009) Historical evolution of the neurotransmission concept. *Journal of Neural Transmission*, 116: 515–33.

Luker, K and Wolfson, D (1999) *Medicines Management for Clinical Nurses.* Oxford: Blackwell Science.

Malkin, B (2008) Are techniques used for intramuscular injection based on research evidence? *Nursing Times*, 104: 48–51.

Mallinger, JB and Lamberti, JS (2006) Clozapine – should race affect prescribing guidelines? *Schizophrenia Research*, 83: 107–8.

Mallinger, JB, Fisher, SG, Brown, T and Lamberti, JS (2006) Racial disparities in the use of second-generation antipsychotics for the treatment of schizophrenia. *Psychiatric Services*, 57: 133–6.

Marder, SR, Mebane, A, Chien, CP, Winslade, WJ, Swan, E and Van Putten, T. (1983) A comparison of patients who refuse and consent to neuroleptic treatment. *American Journal of Psychiatry*, 140 (4): 470–2.

Marom, S, Munitz, H and Jones, PB et al. (2005) Expressed emotion: relevance to rehospitalization in schizophrenia over 7 years. *Schizophrenia Bulletin*, 31, 751–8.

Masimirembwa, CM and Hasler, JA (1997) Genetic polymorphism of drug metabolising enzymes in African populations: implications for the use of neuroleptics and antidepressants. *Brain Research Bulletin*, 44: 561–71.

McCarthy, M, Addington-Hall, J and Altmann, D (1997) The experience of dying with dementia: a retrospective study. *International Journal of Geriatriac Psychiatry*, 12: 404–9.

Mechanic, D, McAlpine, D, Rosenfield, S and Davis, D (1994) Effects of illness attribution and depression on the quality of life among persons with serious mental illness. *Social Science & Medicine*, 39: 155–64.

Moise, P, Schwarzinger, M and Um, MY (2004) *Dementia Care in 9 OECD Countries*. Paris: OECD.

Montgomery, SA, Tobias, K and Zornberg, GL et al. (2006) Efficacy and safety of pregabalin in the treatment of generalized anxiety disorder. *Journal of Clinical Psychiatry*, 67: 771–82.

Muller, DJ, Likhodi, O and Heinz, A (2010) Neural markers of genetic vulnerability to drug addiction. *Current Topics in Behavioural Neuroscience*, 3: 277–99.

Murray, CJ and Lopez, AD (1996) Evidence-based health policy – lessons from the Global Burden of Disease Study. *Science*, 274: 740–3.

Naber, D (1995) A self-rating to measure subjective effects of neuroleptic drugs, relationships to objective psychopathology, quality of life, compliance and other clinical variables. *International Clinical Psychopharmacology*, 10(Suppl. 3): 133–8.

National Institute for Health and Clinical Excellence (NICE) (2007) *Drug Misuse: Opioid detoxification*. London: NICE.

National Institute for Health and Clinical Excellence (NICE) (2009a) *Dementia: Supporting people with dementia and their carers in health and social care*. London: NICE.

National Institute for Health and Clinical Excellence (NICE) (2009b) *Depression: The treatment and management of depression in adults (update)*. London: NICE.

National Institute for Health and Clinical Excellence (NICE) (2009c) *The Guidelines Manual*. London: NICE. Available online at www.nice.org.uk/guidelinesmanual (accessed 5 June 2011).

National Institute for Health and Clinical Excellence (NICE) (2010) *Alcohol Use Disorders: Physical complications*. London: NICE.

National Patient Safety Agency (NPSA) (2007) *Safety in Doses: Medication safety incidents in the NHS*. London: NPSA.

National Patient Safety Agency (NPSA) (2009) *Safety in Doses: Improving the use of medicines in the NHS*. London: NPSA.

National Prescribing Centre (NPC) (1999) Signposts for prescribing nurses. *Prescribing Nurse Bulletin*, 1(1).

Newcomer, JW (2005) Second-generation (atypical) antipsychotics and metabolic effects: a comprehensive literature review. *CNS Drugs*, 19(Suppl. 1): 1–93.

Nursing and Midwifery Council (NMC) (2008a) *The Code: Standards of conduct, performance and ethics for nurses and midwives*. London: NMC.

Nursing and Midwifery Council (NMC) (2008b) *Standards for Medicines Management*. London: NMC.

O'Connell, P, Woodruff, PW and Wright, I et al. (1997) Developmental insanity or dementia praecox: was the wrong concept adopted? *Schizophrenia Research*, 23: 97–106.

Okuma, T (1981) Differential sensitivity to the effects of psychotropic drugs: psychotics vs normals; Asian vs Western populations. *Folia Psychiatrica et Neurologica Japonica*, 35: 79–87.

Olfson, M, Mechanic, D and Hansell, S et al. (2000) Predicting medication noncompliance after hospital discharge among patients with schizophrenia. *Psychiatric Services*, 51: 216–22.

Olfson, M, Marcus, SC and Shaffer, D (2006) Antidepressant drug therapy and suicide in severely depressed children and adults: a case-control study. *Archives of General Psychiatry*, 63: 865–72.

Overstreet, DH, Commissaris, RC and De La Garza, R et al. (2003) Involvement of 5-HT1A receptors in animal tests of anxiety and depression: evidence from genetic models. *Stress*, 6: 101–10.

Phillips, GT, Gossop, M and Bradley, B (1986) The influence of psychological factors on the opiate withdrawal syndrome. *British Journal of Psychiatry*, 149: 235–8.

Plotkin, LL, Bordunovskii, VN, Bazarova, EN and Smirnov, DM (2008) Hepatic protection in patients with generalized purulent peritonitis complicated by sepsis. *Anesteziologiia i Reanimatologiia*, 4: 39–40.

Posternak, MA and Zimmerman, M (2005) Is there a delay in the antidepressant effect? A meta-analysis. *Journal of Clinical Psychiatry*, 66: 148–58.

Pound, P, Britten, N and Morgan, M et al. (2005) Resisting medicines: a synthesis of qualitative studies of medicine taking. *Social Science & Medicine*, 61: 133–55.

Preston, J, O'Neal, J and Talaga, M (2008) *A Handbook of Clinical Psychopharmacology for Therapists*. Oakland, CA: New Harbinger.

Prochaska, JO and Diclemente, CC (1984a) Self change processes, self efficacy and decisional balance across five stages of smoking cessation. *Progress in Clinical and Biological Research*, 156: 131–40.

Prochaska, JO and DiClemente, CC (1984b) *The Transtheoretical Approach: Crossing the traditional boundaries of therapy*. Melbourne, FL: Krieger.

Qurashi, I, Kapur, N and Appleby, L (2006) A prospective study of noncompliance with medication, suicidal ideation, and suicidal behavior in recently discharged psychiatric inpatients. *Archives of Suicide Research*, 10: 61–7.

Ravindran, LN and Stein, MB (2010) The pharmacologic treatment of anxiety disorders: a review of progress. *Journal of Clinical Psychiatry*, 71: 839–54.

Rosa, MA, Marcolin, MA and Elkis, H (2005) Evaluation of the factors interfering with drug treatment compliance among Brazilian patients with schizophrenia. *Revista Brasileira de Psiquiatria*, 27: 178–84.

Rudorfer, MV, Lane, EA and Chang, WH et al. (1984) Desipramine pharmacokinetics in Chinese and Caucasian volunteers. *British Journal of Clinical Pharmacology*, 17: 433–40.

Safran, JD, Muran, JC, Eubanks-Carter, C (2011) Repairing alliance ruptures. *Psychotherapy*, 48(1): 80–7.

Sampson, EL, Gould, V, Lee, D and Blanchard, MR (2006) Differences in care received by patients with and without dementia who died during acute hospital admission: a retrospective case note study. *Age Ageing*, 35: 187–9.

Schatzberg, AF, Haddad, P and Kaplan, EM et al. (1997) Serotonin reuptake inhibitor discontinuation syndrome: a hypothetical definition. *Journal of Clinical Psychiatry*, 58(Suppl. 7): 5–10.

Scher-Svanum, H, Zhu, B and Faries, D et al. (2006) A prospective study of risk factors for nonadherence with antipsychotic medication in the treatment of schizophrenia. *Journal of Clinical Psychiatry*, 67: 1114–23.

Schmitt, R, Gazalle, FK and Lima, MS et al. (2005) The efficacy of antidepressants for generalized anxiety disorder: a systematic review and meta-analysis. *Revista Brasileira Psiquiatria*, 27: 18–24.

Schuckit, MA, Tipp, JE and Reich, T et al. (1995) The histories of withdrawal convulsions and delirium tremens in 1648 alcohol dependent subjects. *Addiction*, 90: 1335–47.

Sellwood, W, Tarrier, N, Quinn, J and Barrowclough, C (2003) The family and compliance in schizophrenia: the influence of clinical variables, relatives' knowledge and expressed emotion. *Psychological Medicine*, 33: 91–6.

Sramek, JJ and Pi, EH (1996) Ethnicity and antidepressant response. *Mount Sinai Journal of Medicine*, 63: 320–5.

Stahl, SM (2008) *Stahl's Essential Psychopharmacology: Neuroscientific basis and practical applications*, 3rd edition. Cambridge: Cambridge University Press.

Stokes, P (2009) Pensioner 'unlawfully killed' by nurse's insulin overdose. *The Daily Telegraph*, 27 March. Available online at www.telegraph.co.uk/news/uknews/5061193 (accessed 1 April 2010).

Strang, J, Marks, I and Dawe, S et al. (1997) Type of hospital setting and treatment outcome with heroin addicts: results from a randomised trial. *British Journal of Psychiatry*, 171: 335–9.

Strickland, TL, Lin, KM and Fu, P et al. (1995) Comparison of lithium ratio between African-American and Caucasian bipolar patients. *Biological Psychiatry*, 37: 325–30.

Strickland, TL, Stein, R and Lin, KM et al. (1997) The pharmacologic treatment of anxiety and depression in African Americans: considerations for the general practitioner. *Archives of Family Medicine*, 6: 371–5.

Swansburg and Swansburg (2002) *Introduction to Management Leadership for Nurse Managers*, 3rd edition. Sudbury, Canada: Jones & Bartlett.

Szasz, T (2007) *Coercion as Cure*. Piscataway, NJ: Transaction Publishers.

Taylor, D, Young, C and Esop, R et al. (2004) Testing for diabetes in hospitalised patients prescribed antipsychotic drugs. *British Journal of Psychiatry*, 185: 152–6.

Taylor, D, Paton, C and Kerwin, R (2007) *The Maudsley Prescribing Guidelines*, 9th edition. London: Informa Healthcare.

Torrey, EF (1994) Violent behavior by individuals with serious mental illness. *Hospital and Community Psychiatry*, 45: 653–62.

Tortora, GL and Derrickson, BH (2008) *Principles of Anatomy and Physiology*, 11th edition. Chicester: Wiley.

Touchon, J, Bergman, H and Bullock, R et al. (2006) Response to rivastigmine or donepezil in Alzheimer's patients with symptoms suggestive of concomitant Lewy body pathology. *Current Medical Research and Opinion*, 22: 49–59.

Trivedi, MH, Rush, AJ and Wisniewski, SR et al. (2006) Evaluation of outcomes with citalopram for depression using measurement-based care in STAR*D: implications for clinical practice. *American Journal of Psychiatry*, 163: 28–40.

Tyrer, P and Murphy, S (1987) The place of benzodiazepines in psychiatric practice. *British Journal of Psychiatry*, 151: 719–23.

Tyrer, P, Casey, PR, Seivewright, H and Seivewright, N (1988) A survey of the treatment of anxiety disorders in general practice. *Postgraduate Medical Journal*, 64(Suppl. 2): 27–31.

van Dyck, CH, Schmitt, FA and Olin, JT (2006) A responder analysis of memantine treatment in patients with Alzheimer disease maintained on donepezil. *American Journal of Geriatric Psychiatry*, 14: 42837.

Van Putten, PT, Crumpton, E and Yale, C (1976) Drug refusal in schizophrenia and the wish to be crazy. *Archives of General Psychiatry*, 33: 1443–6.

Van Putten, PT, May, PR and Marder, SR (1980) Subjective responses to thiothixene and chlorpromazine. *Psychopharmacology Bulletin*, 16: 36–8.

Varner, RV, Ruiz, P and Small, DR (1998) Black and white patients' response to antidepressant treatment for major depression. *Psychiatric Quarterly*, 69: 117–25.

Weeks, KW, Lyne, P and Torrance, C (2000) Written drug dose errors made by students: the threat to clinical effectiveness and the need for a new approach. *Clinical Effectiveness in Nursing*, 4(1): 20–9.

Weiden, P, Shaw, E and Mann, JJ (1986) Causes of neuroleptic noncompliance. *Psychiatric Annals*, 16: 571–5.

Weiden, PJ, Aquila, R, Dalheim, L and Standard, JM (1997) Switching antipsychotic medications. *Journal of Clinical Psychiatry*, 58 (Suppl. 10): 63–72.

Weiden, P, Aquila, R, Emanuel, M and Zygmunt, A (1998) Long-term considerations after switching antipsychotics. *Journal of Clinical Psychiatry*, 59(Suppl. 19): 36–49.

Whiskey, E and Taylor, D (2007) Restarting clozapine after neutropenia: evaluating the possibilities and practicalities. *CNS Drugs*, 21: 25–35.

Wiehl, WO, Hayner, G and Galloway, G (1994) Haight Ashbury Free Clinics' drug detoxification protocols – part 4: alcohol. *Journal of Psychoactive Drugs*, 26: 57–9.

Wilcock, G, Mobius, HJ and Stoffler, A (2002) A double-blind, placebo-controlled multicentre study of memantine in mild to moderate vascular dementia (MMM500). *International Clinical Psychopharmacology*, 17: 297–305.

Williams, DJ (2007) Medication errors. *Journal of the Royal College of Physicians*, 37: 343–6.

Woerner, MG, Alvir, JM and Saltz, BL et al. (1998) Prospective study of tardive dyskinesia in the elderly: rates and risk factors. *American Journal of Psychiatry*, 155: 1521–8.

Workman, B (1999) Safe injection techniques. *Nursing Standard*, 13: 47–53.

World Health Organization (WHO) (2003) *Adherence to Long-term Therapies: Evidence for action*. Geneva: WHO.

Yamada, K, Watanabe, K and Nemoto, N et al. (2006) Prediction of medication noncompliance in outpatients with schizophrenia: 2-year follow-up study. *Psychiatry Research*, 141: 61–9.

Zubin, J and Spring, B (1977) Vulnerability – a new view of schizophrenia. *Journal of Abnormal Psychology*, 86(2): 103–24.

Index